Everything you

need to know

Rheumatology

Caregiver

MARTIN STERLING

Table of contents

Chapter 3: Basic rheumatology care … 31

« In rheumatology, we know that if patience were a joint, it would surely be the most stressed... and sometimes the most rusty! »

Chapter 1

Introduction to Rheumatology

- **Definition and importance of rheumatology**
  Explanation of the specialty and its impact on patients' quality of life.

Rheumatology is a medical specialty that focuses on diseases of the joints, bones, muscles, tendons and ligaments. This field encompasses a wide range of pathologies, from inflammatory conditions such as rheumatoid arthritis to degenerative diseases such as osteoarthritis, and systemic disorders such as lupus. Each rheumatic pathology affects the musculoskeletal system differently, with sometimes profound repercussions on mobility, pain and, inevitably, quality of life.

The role of rheumatology is not simply to diagnose these diseases; it also involves providing tailored, personalized care for each patient, with the aim of minimizing pain and maintaining physical function as effectively as possible. Rheumatic diseases have a direct impact on patients' autonomy. They can lead to significant functional limitations, ranging from difficulty in performing simple daily activities such as standing up or walking, to the inability to carry out social and professional activities. This is why rheumatology treatment is often multidisciplinary, involving both drug treatments (such as anti-inflammatory drugs or biotherapies) and non-drug approaches, such as functional rehabilitation or occupational therapy.

The impact of rheumatology on patients' quality of life is not measured solely by pain management, although this is a priority objective. It's also about restoring self-confidence and giving patients back a sense of control over their bodies and their lives. Chronic illnesses, such as those treated by rheumatology, often have a devastating effect on patients' morale, sometimes plunging them into states of despondency in the face of persistent symptoms. This is where the role of the health-care team, and in particular the nursing auxiliaries, becomes crucial. In addition to physical care, they must provide psychological support and reassurance, and encourage patients to continue treatment and exercise despite the difficulties.

In short, rheumatology is much more than a specialty dealing with joint pain: it is a complex and demanding field, in which the patient's overall well-being is taken into account, both physically and psychologically. This specialty plays a fundamental role in maintaining patients' autonomy and dignity, enabling them to return, as far as possible, to an active and fulfilling life, despite the constraints imposed by their pathologies.

- **Common rheumatological pathologies**
  Rheumatoid arthritis, ankylosing spondylitis, systemic lupus erythematosus, osteoarthritis, gout, etc.

Rheumatology covers a wide range of pathologies, some of which are particularly common and present specific challenges for caregivers and patients alike. Among these, rheumatoid arthritis, ankylosing spondylitis, systemic lupus erythematosus, osteoarthritis and gout top the list for their prevalence and impact on patients' quality of life.

Rheumatoid arthritis is a chronic inflammatory disease that mainly affects small joints, such as those in the hands and feet. It manifests as painful, progressive inflammation of the joints, often leading to deformity and loss of mobility. Unlike osteoarthritis, which is a mechanical wear and tear of the joints, rheumatoid arthritis is an autoimmune disease, in which the immune system mistakenly attacks joint tissue. Patients suffering from this pathology can find their daily activities considerably reduced, ranging from simple discomfort at first to significant disability if the disease is not well controlled. It's a disease that requires careful monitoring and rapid management to avoid irreversible complications.

Ankylosing spondylitis is another inflammatory disease that mainly affects the spine and pelvis. It leads to progressive stiffening of the spinal joints, which may even result in complete fusion of the vertebrae, a condition known as ankylosing spondylitis. The loss of spinal flexibility is often accompanied by chronic back pain, especially on waking, which can greatly affect the patient's mobility and well-being. Young adults, mainly men, are most often affected by this disease, which has a strong psychological impact due to its chronic and disabling nature, especially at an age when physical and professional activities are still central to life.

Systemic lupus erythematosus, commonly known as lupus, is a systemic autoimmune disease that can affect not only the joints, but also the skin, kidneys, heart and even the brain. It's a particularly complex condition, because it manifests itself differently in each patient, with unpredictable flare-ups followed by periods of remission. Lupus patients may experience extreme fatigue, diffuse joint pain and skin problems such as a characteristic butterfly-shaped rash on the face. The unpredictable nature of lupus means that constant care and attention are needed to manage symptoms on a daily basis.

Osteoarthritis, often confused with arthritis, is the most common form of rheumatism, mainly due to wear and tear of articular cartilage. It mainly affects weight-bearing joints, such as the hips and knees, and manifests itself as mechanical pain that intensifies with effort and improves with rest. Unlike inflammatory diseases, osteoarthritis is not directly linked to an attack by the immune system, but rather to the progressive degeneration of joint structures. It is therefore very common in the elderly, but can also occur in younger individuals, especially after joint trauma. Management of osteoarthritis is mainly based on pain management, rehabilitation and, in advanced cases, orthopaedic surgery.

Finally, gout is a metabolic disease characterized by acute inflammatory attacks, often very painful, which mainly affect the joints of the extremities, such as the big toe. It is caused by an accumulation of uric acid crystals in the joints, resulting from poor management of this acid by the kidneys or a diet too rich in purines. Gout attacks usually occur suddenly, often at night, and can make the affected joint red, hot and extremely painful on the slightest touch. Gout is often associated with diseases such as diabetes or hypertension, which further complicates patient management.

These pathologies, although all grouped under the banner of rheumatology, are extremely varied in terms of underlying mechanisms, treatments and impact on patients' lives. Whether inflammatory, degenerative or metabolic, they all share one thing in common: they profoundly alter mobility and daily well-being, requiring holistic management that encompasses not only physical aspects, but also psychological and social dimensions.

- **The caregiver's role in the rheumatology department**
  Collaboration with the nursing team, specific responsibilities and objectives.

Collaboration with the nursing team is at the heart of the work of the rheumatology orderly. Because of the complexity of the pathologies treated, and the diversity of the interventions required, this department is based on a multidisciplinary approach, with each member of the team playing a specific but complementary role. The nursing auxiliary plays a central role in this dynamic, being both the direct link with the patient and an indispensable support for the rest of the care team, comprising doctors, nurses, physiotherapists, occupational therapists and sometimes psychologists.

The responsibilities of the rheumatology orderly are varied and go far beyond basic care. First and foremost, they ensure continuous monitoring of patients' clinical condition. This includes regularly taking vital parameters, assessing pain, and monitoring mobility. Working closely with nurses and doctors, the caregiver is at the forefront of observing the evolution of symptoms and reporting any changes, whether they be worsening pain, the appearance of new inflammation, or increasing difficulty in performing certain movements. This vigilance is crucial, as it enables us to react quickly and appropriately to any complications that may arise.

One of the caregiver's main responsibilities is also to ensure the patient's physical comfort, which in rheumatology can be particularly delicate. Because of the pain and stiffness they cause, rheumatic diseases often restrict patients' mobility. Caregivers must therefore be both attentive and inventive in the way they help patients move around, change position or get out of bed. They may need to use technical aids such as walkers, wheelchairs or special cushions to prevent bedsores. This care, although often perceived as simple, requires great sensitivity to individual patient needs, as well as a perfect knowledge of mobilization techniques to avoid aggravating pain or causing injury.

Another fundamental aspect of the caregiver's role is collaboration in treatment management. Although the administration of certain treatments falls within the remit of nurses and doctors, the caregiver plays a key role in monitoring the effects of treatments, particularly those involving joint pain and inflammation. For example, they are often in charge of applying local treatments such as dressings, applying hot or cold compresses to relieve pain or reduce swelling, as well as helping patients comply with their medication regimens. In the case of **biotherapies** or other specific treatments such as subcutaneous injections, the caregiver ensures extra vigilance with regard to side effects, immediately reporting any abnormal signs.

The objectives of the rheumatology caregiver are therefore manifold, but they all revolve around one central goal: to improve patients' quality of life, while facilitating their recovery and preventing complications. This involves not only alleviating physical pain, but also encouraging patients to regain a degree of autonomy, even in the smallest daily activities. The caregiver often plays a key role in functional rehabilitation, collaborating with physiotherapists to help patients perform rehabilitation exercises, or helping set up adapted techniques for movements as simple as dressing or washing.

Finally, collaboration with the care team also extends to the psychological and social field. Rheumatic diseases, particularly the chronic forms, can have a considerable impact on patients' morale. Through their daily contact with patients, caregivers often play a role in providing moral support, active listening and mediation between the various healthcare professionals and the patient. They can help to allay fears or frustrations, explain medical instructions more clearly, or simply be a reassuring presence at difficult times. It is this close relationship, coupled with close collaboration with the entire care team, that enables the caregiver to have a significant impact on patients' overall well-being.

Chapter 2

Anatomy and Physiopathology of the Musculoskeletal System

- **Anatomy of joints, bones and muscles**
  Description of structures and their functions.

The musculoskeletal system is a marvel of biological engineering, composed of multiple structures that work in harmony to enable movement, support the body and protect vital organs. This system is based on a close interaction between bones, joints, muscles, tendons and ligaments, each with a very specific and essential function.

Bones form the backbone of the human body. They form the skeleton, a rigid yet dynamic structure that both supports the body and protects the internal organs. Bones are much more than just structural parts: they are also the site of blood cell production in the bone marrow, and play an important role in the storage of minerals, such as calcium and phosphorus, required for many physiological functions. Bones vary in shape and size, from long bones like the femur to flatter, more protective bones like the skull, each adapted to its precise role.

Joints, meanwhile, are the junction points between bones. They enable movement and are crucial to the body's flexibility and mobility. There are several types of joint, some of which are immobile, such as those in the skull, and others which allow a wide range of movement, such as the synovial joints found in the shoulders, knees and hips. These joints are lubricated by synovial fluid, a viscous substance that reduces friction between the bones and enables fluid movement. Cartilage, another key component of joints, acts as a shock absorber, protecting the bony ends from impact and wear.

Muscles are the motors of movement. Attached to the bones by tendons, muscles contract to generate the force needed to move bony structures. There are three types of muscle in the human body, but those primarily involved in movement are the skeletal muscles. They function voluntarily, under the control of our central nervous system, enabling us to walk, run, lift objects or perform fine gestures such as writing or playing an instrument. Muscle contraction relies on a complex sliding mechanism between muscle fibers which, although microscopic, is capable of producing movements of great amplitude.

Tendons, which connect muscles to bones, are strong, flexible fibrous structures. They are essential for transmitting the force generated by muscles to bones, enabling movement. Without tendons, muscles could not exert their action on the skeleton. These structures are designed to withstand great tension, but they can be vulnerable to wear and tear, particularly under conditions of overwork or inflammation.

Ligaments, on the other hand, are bands of connective tissue that link bones together at the joints. Their main role is to stabilize joints, limiting their range of movement and preventing excessive displacement that could damage joint structures. Ligaments are particularly important in complex, mobile joints such as the knees and shoulders, where they help prevent dislocations and sprains.

All these structures - bones, joints, muscles, tendons and ligaments - work in synergy to ensure the body's mobility and stability. When this system functions correctly, it enables a wide range of movements, from simple maintenance of standing posture to more complex and precise actions. However, any disturbance in any of these structures, whether caused by disease, injury or degeneration, can lead to pain, loss of function and impaired quality of life. This is why a detailed understanding of these structures and their functions is essential for healthcare professionals, particularly in specialties such as rheumatology, where disorders of the musculoskeletal system are at the heart of management.

- **Pathological mechanisms of rheumatic diseases**
  Inflammatory, degenerative and autoimmune processes.
Inflammatory, degenerative and autoimmune processes represent three major pathological mechanisms affecting the musculoskeletal system, each with specific causes and

consequences, but all leading to significant alterations in joint, muscle and bone function.

Inflammatory processes are at the heart of many rheumatic diseases. Inflammation is the body's natural response to aggression, whether infection, trauma or irritation. However, in chronic inflammatory diseases such as rheumatoid arthritis, this response becomes inappropriate and self-sustaining. Instead of protecting the body, inflammation becomes excessively prolonged, damaging joints. Immune system cells invade joint tissue, releasing inflammatory substances that cause progressive destruction of cartilage and bone. This inflammatory process leads to pain, swelling, loss of mobility and, ultimately, joint deformity. Patients suffering from these diseases often experience morning stiffness and intense fatigue, in addition to persistent joint pain. Managing inflammation is therefore a central objective in the management of inflammatory rheumatic diseases, with the use of anti-inflammatory drugs, immunosuppressants or biotherapies aimed at modulating the immune response.

Degenerative processes, on the other hand, are at the root of diseases such as osteoarthritis. Unlike chronic inflammation, here the problem lies in the gradual wear and tear of joint structures, particularly cartilage. Cartilage, which normally acts as a shock absorber between bones, gradually deteriorates under the effect of repeated mechanical stress or aging. With the loss of cartilage, bones begin to rub directly against each other, resulting in pain, stiffness and loss of function. Osteoarthritis often affects weight-bearing joints such as the knees and hips, making simple activities such as walking or climbing stairs extremely difficult. This degenerative process is often irreversible, but can be slowed by interventions designed to reduce the mechanical overload on the joints, such as functional rehabilitation or the use of joint prostheses in the most advanced cases. Although not directly inflammatory, joint degeneration can lead to episodes of reactive inflammation when fragments of worn cartilage irritate the joint.

Autoimmune processes are another key category of rheumatic disease. In these pathologies, the immune system, normally responsible for defending the body against infection and foreign agents, mistakenly begins to attack healthy tissue. Rheumatoid arthritis and systemic lupus erythematosus are two emblematic examples of this mechanism. In these diseases, immune cells identify joints, skin or other organs as targets to be eliminated. This leads to chronic inflammation and progressive damage to the affected tissues. Unlike acute inflammation caused by infection or injury, autoimmune inflammation is perpetuated by abnormalities in the immune system itself, making it particularly difficult to control. Lupus, for example, can affect several organ systems in addition to the joints, including the kidneys, heart and nervous system, making management of the disease extremely complex.

These autoimmune processes, in addition to causing pain and joint damage, also have a significant impact on patients' overall health. They can lead to chronic fatigue, skin rashes, heart and kidney problems, and significantly affect quality of life. Management of these autoimmune diseases often relies on long-term treatments aimed at regulating the immune system to limit damage to joints and organs. This may include the use of corticosteroids, immunosuppressive drugs, or biotherapies targeting specific immune system compounds involved in the inflammatory process.

In short, these three mechanisms - inflammation, degeneration and autoimmunity - do not occur in isolation. They may coexist in the same patient, exacerbating the progression of the disease. For example, chronic inflammation can accelerate cartilage degeneration, while autoimmune disease can lead to recurrent inflammatory flare-ups. Understanding these processes enables caregivers to tailor treatments to the underlying cause, and to offer more targeted and effective management, with the ultimate aim of improving patients' quality of life by limiting pain, preserving joint function, and slowing the progression of lesions.

- **The impact of pathologies on patients' mobility and quality of life**
  Functional limitations, chronic pain and associated comorbidities.

Rheumatic diseases often lead to significant **functional limitations**, profoundly impacting patients' daily lives. These limitations arise mainly from joint stiffness, loss of mobility, and pain affecting joints, muscles and tendons. For example, a patient with rheumatoid arthritis may have difficulty performing gestures as simple as turning a doorknob, buttoning a shirt or getting up from a chair. Similarly, a person with advanced osteoarthritis may find it painful to walk, climb stairs, or even stand for long periods. These functional restrictions are not limited to everyday gestures, but also affect patients' ability to maintain a professional or social activity, which can lead to progressive loss of autonomy and isolation.

At the same time, **chronic pain** is a constant burden for people with rheumatic diseases. Unlike acute pain, which signals a one-off injury or trauma, chronic pain in rheumatology is persistent and results from an ongoing inflammatory or degenerative process. This pain may vary in intensity, but it is often permanently present, fluctuating, and particularly exacerbated during movement or effort. This contributes to a vicious circle: pain limits mobility, leading to a loss of joint and muscle flexibility, further exacerbating pain when the patient attempts to mobilize. This pain, sometimes diffuse and difficult to localize, can also disrupt sleep, leading to increased fatigue and making day-to-day symptom management even more difficult. Beyond the physical discomfort, chronic pain also has a significant psychological impact, leading to depression, anxiety and feelings of helplessness.

Comorbidities associated with rheumatic diseases further complicate the clinical picture. These pathologies are not limited to the joints; they often have systemic repercussions and are frequently associated with other health disorders. For example, the immobility of osteoarthritis can increase the risk of cardiovascular disease, such as hypertension or heart failure, as patients become less physically active. What's more, taking certain treatments, such as corticosteroids or non-steroidal anti-inflammatory drugs (NSAIDs), can have long-term side-effects, such as high blood pressure, osteoporosis or gastrointestinal disorders.

In inflammatory diseases such as rheumatoid arthritis or systemic lupus erythematosus, comorbidities are even more numerous. These autoimmune diseases affect not only the joints, but also other organs, creating multi-organ complications. For example, lupus patients are at greater risk of developing kidney problems, skin disorders and heart disease. In addition, the chronic systemic inflammation associated with rheumatoid arthritis is associated with an increased risk of cardiovascular disease, osteoporosis and metabolic syndrome. The presence of these comorbidities makes disease management more complex, and calls for comprehensive, multidisciplinary management.

Patients often have to juggle several treatments simultaneously, each aimed at a specific condition. For example, a patient may receive anti-inflammatory drugs to relieve joint pain, medications to control blood pressure, and treatments to manage type 2 diabetes which may be exacerbated by steroids. This multiplicity of treatments increases the risk of drug interactions, confusion and poor compliance, especially in the elderly.

Finally, psychological comorbidities such as anxiety and depression are common in patients with chronic rheumatic diseases. The constant burden of pain, the uncertainty of disease progression, and the progressive loss of autonomy create significant stress. Patients may feel helpless in the face of unpredictable inflammatory flare-ups or the slow but inexorable progression of joint degeneration. This psychological stress must be taken into account in the overall management of the patient, as it can alter pain perception and further exacerbate functional limitations.

Chapter 3

Basic Rheumatology Care

- **Clinical monitoring and follow-up of rheumatology patients**
  Vital parameters, pain, mobility assessment.

As part of rheumatology patient follow-up, observation and monitoring of **vital parameters**, **pain** and **mobility** are essential aspects in assessing disease progression, treatment efficacy and overall patient well-being. These elements form the pillars of daily care, and regular monitoring enables therapeutic interventions to be adjusted appropriately.

Vital parameters are fundamental measurements that reflect the patient's general condition. In rheumatology, although diseases mainly affect the joints, systemic damage can also occur, which is why it is crucial to monitor indicators such as body temperature, blood pressure, heart rate and oxygen saturation. For example, a persistent fever may signal an infection, a frequent complication in patients on immunosuppressants for inflammatory conditions such as rheumatoid arthritis or systemic lupus erythematosus. Similarly, an increase in blood pressure may be a sign of a complication linked to certain treatments, such as corticosteroids, or to an associated comorbidity. Monitoring these vital parameters not only helps prevent complications, but also detects signs of deterioration in general health, sometimes necessitating urgent medical intervention.

Pain management and assessment are also central to the care of rheumatology patients. Pain, whether acute or chronic, is a ubiquitous symptom in these pathologies. The intensity, location and type of pain (inflammatory, mechanical, neuropathic) must be assessed regularly to better understand its origin and adapt treatment. Patients suffering from rheumatoid arthritis, for example, often report inflammatory pain, characterized by a sensation of heat, swelling and stiffness, especially in the morning. In contrast, osteoarthritis patients tend to describe mechanical pain, which intensifies after exertion and improves with rest. Pain assessment must therefore be detailed and continuous, using tools such as the numerical pain scale, or more comprehensive questionnaires that provide a clearer picture of the impact of pain on daily life. By taking into account both the physical and psychological aspects of pain, caregivers can better adapt treatments, whether they involve medication, rehabilitation techniques or psychological support.

Mobility assessment is another essential component, as rheumatic diseases primarily affect movement capacity. Mobility can be compromised on a number of levels: by pain, by joint stiffness or by muscle weakness. Mobility assessment involves more than simply observing whether or not a patient can move; it involves a detailed analysis of how he or she performs specific movements, such as getting up from a chair, walking a short distance, climbing stairs or performing fine tasks like opening a bottle or handling objects. This assessment also includes joint range of motion, which may be restricted by inflammation or degeneration, and muscle strength, which may weaken due to pain or lack of exercise.

The caregiver plays a key role in this assessment. By observing patients' movements on a daily basis and noting any difficulties they encounter, they help to adjust rehabilitation programs and identify when further intervention is required, whether by a physiotherapist or an occupational therapist. The caregiver can also encourage patients to use technical aids such as canes, walkers or orthoses to facilitate movement and preserve as much autonomy as possible. Regular monitoring of mobility helps prevent complications associated with immobility, such as bedsores or muscle atrophy, and encourages active rehabilitation.

- **Hygiene and skin care for patients with rheumatic diseases**
  Precautions to avoid skin complications linked to immobility.

Prolonged immobility, often encountered in patients with rheumatic diseases, exposes the skin to a high risk of complications, in particular the formation of pressure sores. These skin lesions result from the prolonged compression of soft tissue between a rigid surface, such as a bed or chair, and the underlying bones. This continuous compression reduces local blood circulation, depriving the skin and surrounding tissues of oxygen and essential nutrients, leading to progressive cell death and wound formation. Preventing these complications is a top priority in the care of immobilized patients, and requires constant attention and specific measures.

Regular mobilization of patients is the first essential preventive measure to avoid pressure sores and other skin complications associated with immobility. It's important to reposition bedridden or wheelchair-bound patients at least every two hours to relieve pressure on at-risk areas such as the sacrum, heels, hips and elbows. Frequent changes of position allow blood to circulate more freely in compressed areas, reducing the risk of tissue ischemia. The caregiver, often in the front line of care, plays a key role in this regular mobilization, using lifting techniques or adjusting cushions and supports to redistribute pressure points.

The **use of specific mattresses and cushions** is another essential precaution to prevent skin complications. Dynamic air mattresses, which regularly change pressure points by inflating and deflating certain sections, are particularly effective for patients confined to bed for long periods. Similarly, foam or gel positioning cushions are used to relieve pressure on vulnerable areas when the patient is in a wheelchair. These devices are designed to distribute pressure more evenly and reduce the risk of skin lesions. The caregiver must ensure that these devices are used correctly, adjusted according to the patient's needs, and regularly inspected to ensure their effectiveness.

At the same time, meticulous attention must be paid **to skin hygiene and hydration**. Clean, well-moisturized skin is less vulnerable to external aggressions and lesions. Cleansing should be carried out regularly, avoiding excessive friction that could irritate fragile skin. After cleansing, the application of suitable moisturizers helps maintain the skin barrier in good condition, preventing dryness and cracking. Particular attention should be paid to areas prone to maceration, such as skin folds or areas of prolonged contact with medical devices, as excessive moisture weakens the skin and increases the risk of pressure sores.

Rigorous monitoring of skin condition is another crucial aspect of preventing skin complications. The caregiver must inspect the patient's skin daily, especially in pressure areas, looking for early signs of injury. Redness that does not disappear with pressure is often the first sign of an incipient pressure sore. If these signs are spotted early, preventive interventions can be put in place, such as changing the patient's position or using extra protection, to prevent the lesion from progressing. A daily assessment can also identify other skin problems, such as irritations, sores or infections, which could further complicate the patient's condition.

Nutrition also plays a fundamental role in skin health and the prevention of skin complications. Immobilized patients are often at risk of malnutrition, which weakens skin resistance and slows wound healing. The provision of proteins, vitamins (particularly C and E) and minerals such as zinc is essential to maintain skin integrity and promote tissue regeneration. The nursing auxiliary, in collaboration with dieticians and nurses, must ensure that patients receive a balanced and sufficient diet, or nutritional supplements if necessary, to support their skin and body in the prevention of pressure sores.

Finally, **ongoing training for caregivers** in pressure sore prevention techniques and specific skin care is essential to ensure optimal care for immobilized patients. With regular training in new technologies and best practices, caregivers are better equipped to spot signs of skin deterioration and intervene early and appropriately.

- **Mobility assistance and pain management**
  Use of technical aids, physiotherapy and psychological support.

In rheumatology, the use of **technical aids**, **physiotherapy** and **psychological support** form a coherent and indispensable whole to improve patients' quality of life. These complementary approaches not only alleviate physical symptoms such as pain and functional limitations, but also meet the emotional and psychological needs of patients, who are often weakened by the progression of their disease.

The **use of technical aids** plays a central role in the management of rheumatic diseases, particularly when patients' mobility is impaired by pain, joint stiffness or muscle weakness. These devices, such as canes, walkers, wheelchairs and orthoses, are designed to compensate for physical limitations while promoting patient autonomy. For example, a person suffering from osteoarthritis of the hips or knees may benefit from a cane to relieve some of the weight borne by their joints when walking. Similarly, patients suffering from rheumatoid arthritis can use splints to stabilize affected joints and reduce pain during movement.

The caregiver, in conjunction with the physiotherapist and occupational therapist, plays a crucial role in adjusting and learning to use these technical aids. They must not only ensure that the equipment is adapted to the patient's specific needs, but also that the patient is comfortable in its day-to-day use. This sometimes involves training the patient in simple but essential gestures, such as the correct way to use a cane or to get out of a wheelchair without risking a fall. These technical aids not only help reduce the pain and fatigue associated with movement, but also preserve a sense of independence, which is fundamental to patients' psychological well-being.

At the same time, **physiotherapy** is an essential pillar in the rehabilitation of patients suffering from rheumatic diseases. The role of the physiotherapist is to restore or maintain joint mobility, strengthen weakened muscles, and prevent stiffness or deformity that may result from immobility or pain. Physiotherapy is not just a series of physical exercises; it is also a gentle therapeutic approach that adapts to each patient's abilities and limitations. In inflammatory diseases, for example, such as ankylosing spondylitis, where the spine gradually loses its flexibility, the physiotherapist will propose specific mobility and stretching exercises to prevent ankylosis (joint stiffness) and maintain joint flexibility as far as possible.

Physiotherapy sessions are also essential to strengthen the muscles that surround and support the joints. Improving muscle strength reduces the load directly exerted on the joints, helping to reduce pain and improve overall function. In addition, physiotherapy plays a preventive role in avoiding secondary complications associated with prolonged immobility, such as muscle loss or atrophy. The caregiver actively collaborates with the physiotherapist to encourage patients to perform their exercises regularly and to integrate these movements into their daily lives, whether in hospital or at home.

Finally, **psychological support** is a fundamental component in the care of patients with chronic rheumatic diseases. Living with constant pain, physical limitations and sometimes visible deformities can have a considerable impact on self-esteem and mental health. Diseases such as rheumatoid arthritis or systemic lupus erythematosus, which can lead to unpredictable and disabling flare-ups, often plunge patients into a state of anxiety or discouragement when faced with the uncertainty of their condition. Fear of gradual loss of autonomy, coupled with chronic pain, can also lead to depression.

By being in direct daily contact with patients, caregivers are often the first to spot signs of emotional distress. By actively listening, offering encouragement and validating patients' feelings, they help to lighten the psychological burden of illness. Sometimes, simply acknowledging the difficulty of living with chronic pain or reduced mobility helps patients feel understood and supported. This day-to-day support can also be reinforced by collaboration with psychologists, who provide specialized help in managing the emotional aspects of the disease, particularly when symptoms of depression or anxiety appear.

Support groups and group therapies are also valuable resources for patients with chronic illnesses. Sharing one's experience with other patients facing similar challenges helps to break down isolation and reinforce the feeling of not being alone in the face of illness. This kind of psychological support can have both emotional and physical benefits, as higher morale often improves pain perception and encourages greater participation in care.

- **Preventing pressure sores and other complications associated with immobility**
  Regular positioning and mobilization techniques.

Regular settling and mobilization techniques are essential practices in the care of patients, particularly those suffering from rheumatic diseases or other pathologies that restrict mobility. These techniques aim to prevent complications associated with prolonged immobility, such as pressure sores, contractures and muscular atrophy, while ensuring patient comfort and preserving maximum autonomy.

Correct patient positioning is the first aspect to consider in preventing complications. When a patient is bedridden or in a chair for long periods, it is crucial to ensure that the body is correctly positioned to avoid pressure points, reduce muscle tension and promote good blood circulation. For example, in a bed, the patient should be positioned so that the spine is aligned, with adequate support for the hips, knees and ankles. Cushions can be placed under the knees or between the legs to maintain correct alignment and prevent joints locking into uncomfortable or potentially damaging positions.

In addition, for patients suffering from joint pain, such as those with rheumatoid arthritis, special attention must be paid to sensitive areas. Special cushions or support devices can be used to relieve pressure on painful joints, such as hips or shoulders, and to prevent excessive friction that could aggravate inflammation or cause sores. These installation techniques are designed to offer maximum comfort, while reducing the risk of skin or musculoskeletal complications.

However, **proper installation** alone is not enough to guarantee patient health and well-being. **Regular mobilization** is just as important. Repositioning the patient every two hours, for example, is a crucial measure in preventing the formation of pressure sores, which occur when certain areas of the body remain under prolonged pressure. Immobilized patients, especially those unable to mobilize themselves, require careful monitoring and assistance to change position regularly. This may include simple movements, such as moving from a supine to a semi-seated position, or turning the patient from side to side in bed. These position changes not only relieve pressure areas, but also promote better blood circulation and prevent numbness or pain associated with prolonged immobility.

Mobilization is not just about changing position. It also involves **passive** and **active mobilization** techniques. Passive mobilization is particularly useful for patients with limited range of motion or who are unable to move on their own. In this method, the caregiver helps the patient perform joint movements, such as bending and extending the knees or arms, without the patient having to exert any effort. This keeps joints supple, prevents stiffness and encourages blood circulation. Active mobilization, on the other hand, involves the patient's active participation in movements, even if he or she needs assistance to carry them out. This type of mobilization strengthens muscles, improves coordination, and stimulates the patient's functional autonomy.

It is also important to consider **mobilization** techniques **when lifting a patient**. Helping a patient move from a sitting to a standing position, or from a chair to a bed, requires appropriate techniques to avoid injury to both patient and caregiver. The use of technical aids such as patient lifts, support bars or transfer belts can facilitate these movements while ensuring safety. By applying appropriate lifting and transfer techniques, the caregiver can encourage the patient to participate as much as possible, thus reducing the feeling of dependence and promoting autonomy.

Finally, regular mobilization also has a positive psychological impact on the patient. The simple fact of being able to move around, even with assistance, or to change position regularly can reduce anxiety and the feeling of being "stuck" in the same position. This helps to improve morale, and better mobility is often associated with a more positive perception of overall health. What's more, mobilization helps prevent complications associated with immobility, such as respiratory infections or circulatory problems, which can arise when the patient remains inactive for too long.

Chapter 4

Patient support

- **Active listening and communication with rheumatology patients**
  The importance of a trusting relationship, taking pain and fears into account.

The **relationship of trust** between patient and healthcare team is a fundamental pillar of chronic disease management, particularly in rheumatology, where pain, functional limitations and the uncertainty of disease progression are daily realities for patients. This relationship, built up over time, plays a crucial role not only in adherence to treatment, but also in the patient's psychological and emotional well-being. When patients feel understood, listened to and respected, they are more inclined to express their needs and concerns, and to actively collaborate in their own healing process.

The importance of this **trust** can be seen first and foremost in pain management, which is often omnipresent in patients with rheumatic diseases. Pain, whether acute or chronic, has a major impact on quality of life. But the perception of this pain varies from one individual to another, and depends on many factors, including the emotional support received. When the caregiver takes the time to listen to descriptions of pain, without minimizing its intensity or frequency, this allows the patient to feel heard and taken seriously. This validation of symptoms is essential, as it shows the patient that their suffering is recognized, which is often the first step towards relief, whether physical or psychological.

Managing patients' pain involves much more than simply administering medication. It also means adapting care and daily activities to the pain levels reported. For example, caregivers can adjust the way they help a patient get up or turn around in bed, paying attention to movements that might exacerbate pain. Simply asking regular questions about pain and suggesting adjustments or alternatives reinforces the relationship of trust. It shows the patient that his or her comfort is a priority, and that he or she can count on the care team to adjust care to his or her real needs.

At the same time, **taking the** patient's **fears into account** is just as crucial. Rheumatic diseases, particularly chronic forms such as rheumatoid arthritis or ankylosing spondylitis, are often accompanied by a series of fears: fear of worsening symptoms, fear of loss of autonomy, and fear of future pain. These fears, although they may seem abstract, are realities deeply felt by patients and influence their state of mind on a daily basis. Not recognizing or ignoring them can lead to emotional isolation, with patients feeling misunderstood or abandoned in the face of the seriousness of their situation.

The caregiver, by being close to the patient, has a unique role to play in accepting and managing these fears. They are often the first to perceive signs of anxiety or doubt in the patient. By creating a reassuring environment, where the patient feels free to express his or her anxieties without judgment, the caregiver helps to defuse these fears to some extent. Simply asking open-ended questions, listening actively, and responding with empathy can help reduce the stress felt by the patient. This does not necessarily mean superficial reassurance, but rather accompanying the patient in understanding his or her illness, providing clear information and being there to answer questions.

Fears about the future - such as the progression of the disease or the fear of becoming dependent - also need to be addressed sensitively. Explaining to the patient the different possible stages of the disease, the long-term treatment options, and the resources available to help them remain as independent as possible can allay some of these anxieties. Transparency, combined with constant support, helps to reduce uncertainty, which in turn helps to strengthen the relationship of trust.

Finally, it's important to recognize that this relationship of trust is built not only around the technical aspects of care, but also through the **human presence** of the caregiver. Being available, even for simple gestures or daily exchanges, strengthens this connection. A smile, a word of encouragement or a moment of listening can have a significant impact on a patient's morale. This feeling of being supported, both physically and emotionally, helps patients to overcome difficult moments and face their illness with greater serenity.

- **Psychological support for patients with chronic illnesses**
  The importance of empathy and support in the face of daily challenges.

Empathy and **support** are essential elements in the care of patients with chronic illnesses, particularly in rheumatology, where the daily challenges are numerous and deeply rooted in the reality of pain, fatigue and functional limitations. These illnesses, often invisible to others, confront patients with constant inner suffering, which is not limited solely to physical pain, but also extends to psychological and emotional dimensions. In this context, the empathy and support offered by caregivers play a crucial role in alleviating this burden and improving patients' quality of life.

Empathy enables caregivers to put themselves in the patient's shoes, to imagine how he or she feels about chronic pain, loss of mobility, or the uncertain course of the disease. It's much more than a simple act of sympathy or benevolence; it's a genuine emotional understanding of the experience of illness, enabling us to respond appropriately to each patient's specific needs. By being empathetic, the caregiver recognizes that each patient experiences their illness differently, and that the psychological impact of pain or loss of autonomy can be just as important as the physical symptoms themselves. This understanding makes it possible to personalize care and respond to the patient's emotional expectations, strengthening the relationship of trust and fostering greater cooperation in treatment.

Empathy manifests itself in many aspects of care. For example, when a patient expresses pain or frustration with physical limitations, attentive listening and non-judgment are strong signs of empathy. By taking the time to listen, even at moments when speech seems simple or banal, the caregiver shows that he or she recognizes the reality of the challenges the patient faces on a daily basis. This active listening creates a space where patients feel safe to express their emotions, fears or anxieties, without fear of being misunderstood or minimized. This emotional support is all the more valuable as patients with chronic illnesses can sometimes feel isolated, even when surrounded by loved ones, because their pain or fatigue is difficult to share or explain.

Support with **everyday challenges** is just as important as empathy. Rheumatology patients face constant difficulties in accomplishing simple tasks once taken for granted, such as getting up, getting dressed or walking. These everyday gestures become trials in themselves, and the patient can quickly feel overwhelmed by the accumulation of small victories needed to simply function day by day. The caregiver's role here is fundamental: to offer both physical support, through adapted gestures, and emotional support, by encouraging the patient not to be discouraged by these challenges.

This support takes the form of concrete actions. For example, helping a patient to use technical aids, showing them how to adjust their environment to make it more functional, or suggesting solutions to reduce the fatigue or pain associated with certain daily activities. This support is not only practical, but also reinforces the patient's confidence in his or her ability to regain a certain degree of autonomy. Even if the disease limits their movements or abilities, patients can feel that they retain control over their daily lives, thanks to the caregiver's benevolent, proactive assistance.

Nor should we underestimate the importance of **moral support** in the face of fluctuating illness. Rheumatic diseases are often characterized by flare-ups and remissions, creating a sense of unpredictability that can be mentally exhausting for the patient. Uncertainty about the future, periods of increased pain or sudden limitations can lead to profound discouragement. At such times, empathy alone is not enough; what's needed is active support, a constant presence that reminds the patient that he's not alone in his struggle. Encouragement, small gestures and accompanying the patient through every stage of his or her treatment all help to boost morale and give the patient the energy needed to face these difficult moments.

Psychological support is particularly crucial in helping patients accept their condition and cope with the upheavals it entails. By collaborating with psychologists or therapists, the caregiver can direct the patient towards additional resources, but his or her own role remains paramount: to be a figure of trust, on whom the patient knows he or she can rely on a daily basis. The caregiver's emotional support often helps to alleviate the anxiety, depression and loneliness that often accompany chronic illness.

- **Support for patients at the end of life or in critical phases**
  Palliative care, pain management and family support.

The **palliative approach** in rheumatology, as in other fields of medicine, focuses on supporting patients suffering from progressive chronic diseases with an uncertain or guarded prognosis. Unlike a curative approach, which aims to cure, the palliative approach focuses on quality of life, seeking to relieve pain and meet patients' physical, emotional and spiritual needs. This approach is particularly crucial for patients in the advanced stages of severe rheumatic diseases, or when treatments are no longer able to halt the progression of the disease. It involves not only careful symptom management, but also holistic support that embraces both patient and family.

Pain management is one of the main thrusts of this approach. In chronic rheumatic diseases, pain often becomes a daily companion, fluctuating in intensity but omnipresent. In palliative care, the aim is to reduce this pain as much as possible, enabling the patient to regain a certain degree of comfort, while respecting his or her wishes and life priorities. This is achieved not only through drug treatments, but also through non-pharmacological approaches. Pain medication, whether mild like paracetamol or more potent like opioids, is used according to the intensity of the pain and the patient's needs. Dose titration and continuous adaptation of treatments are essential to achieve a balance between pain relief and maintenance of optimal quality of life, without undue side effects.

However, **pain management** does not rely solely on medication. In palliative care, techniques such as massage, relaxation, thermotherapy (application of heat or cold), and even gentle mobilization can play an important role in relieving joint or muscle pain. Complementary approaches, such as music therapy or guided meditation, can also offer psychological relief by helping the patient to focus on something other than the pain, while promoting general soothing.

In addition to pain management, the palliative approach places great importance on **emotional and psychological support**, both for the patient and his or her family. When a patient with a rheumatic disease enters the palliative phase, he or she is often confronted with feelings of loss, fear and uncertainty about the future. The caregiver, in liaison with the multidisciplinary team, becomes a key figure in this delicate period, offering attentive listening and a reassuring presence. Sometimes, the simple presence of an empathetic caregiver, ready to listen to the patient's concerns, answer their questions or support them in moments of doubt, can bring immense comfort.

Family support is another essential aspect of the palliative approach. Those close to a patient in the advanced stages of a chronic illness often experience distress too, feeling powerless in the face of their loved one's suffering. They may experience feelings of guilt, sadness or frustration, and need support in understanding the progression of the disease and the options available to relieve their loved one. Here, the caregiver plays the role of mediator between the medical team and the family, clearly explaining proposed interventions, reassuring them about the care being provided, and offering a space for open dialogue where loved ones' concerns can be expressed and heard.

What's more, the palliative approach involves preparation for the end of life, a subject that is often difficult for families to broach. Caregivers must show great sensitivity and delicacy in accompanying loved ones in this process, while respecting the patient's wishes. This may involve decisions about limiting aggressive treatments, organizing care at home, or respecting the patient's wishes regarding his or her final moments. By helping the family to better understand this process, the healthcare team reduces the stress and anxiety associated with uncertainty, and enables loved ones to concentrate on providing emotional support to their loved one.

Family support does not stop at managing the medical aspects. It also includes support in grieving and coping with loss. As the end of life approaches, families need to know that they are not alone at this difficult time. By maintaining an open dialogue, explaining the changes that may occur, and providing ongoing psychological support, the care team helps loved ones face this transitional period with greater serenity. After the death, follow-up care can be offered to help families through the bereavement process, either through support groups or individual interviews with psychologists.

Chapter 5

Pain Management

- **Types of pain in rheumatology**

Inflammatory, mechanical and neuropathic pain.

Inflammatory, **mechanical** and **neuropathic pain** are three distinct types of pain, each with specific underlying mechanisms, different manifestations, and requiring tailored therapeutic approaches. In rheumatology, the distinction between these types of pain is crucial in guiding treatment and offering patients effective, lasting relief.

Inflammatory pain is often present in chronic rheumatic diseases, such as rheumatoid arthritis or ankylosing spondylitis. This type of pain results from an inflammatory process, where the immune system mistakenly attacks the joints, causing inflammation of the tissues surrounding the joint. This inflammation leads to swelling, redness, heat in the joint and intense pain. Inflammatory pain tends to be most marked at rest and upon awakening, particularly in the morning, with joint stiffness lasting several hours before improving over the course of the day as the patient moves. Far from aggravating the pain, movement tends to relieve it progressively, unlike other forms of pain. Treatment of inflammatory pain is based on the use of non-steroidal anti-inflammatory drugs (NSAIDs), corticosteroids or biotherapies to reduce the inflammatory response and, consequently, alleviate pain.

Mechanical pain, on the other hand, is linked to a degenerative process, in which wear and tear of joints, muscles or tendons plays a central role. The most common example is osteoarthritis, a degenerative condition in which articular cartilage gradually wears away, leaving bones rubbing directly against each other. This friction causes pain that is particularly pronounced during movement or exertion, such as walking, climbing stairs or lifting objects. Unlike inflammatory pain, mechanical pain generally improves with rest, but intensifies with activity. It is often localized in weight-bearing joints, such as the knees or hips, where wear is most pronounced. A distinctive feature of this form of pain is that patients may feel cracking or creaking in the joints during movement. Management of mechanical pain includes weight management to reduce pressure on the joints, rehabilitation exercises to strengthen the surrounding muscles, and the use of analgesics to relieve pain. In some advanced cases, surgical intervention, such as joint replacement, may be required to restore joint function.

Neuropathic pain, on the other hand, is completely different in nature from inflammatory or mechanical pain. It results from a lesion or dysfunction of the nervous system, leading to a sensation of pain without external pain stimulation. In other words, the nervous system sends abnormal pain signals to the brain, even in the absence of direct or immediate tissue damage. This type of pain is often described as burning, electric shocks, tingling or numbness. In rheumatology, neuropathic pain can be associated with conditions such as ankylosing spondylitis, where nerves may be compressed by fused vertebrae or inflammation of the tissue around vertebral joints. It can also occur after nerve damage due to surgery or joint trauma. Unlike inflammatory or mechanical pain, neuropathic pain is often more difficult to treat, as it does not respond well to conventional analgesic treatments. Specific medications for neuropathic pain, such as anticonvulsants or certain antidepressants, are often used to modulate nerve activity and attenuate these abnormal sensations. Complementary approaches, such as transcutaneous electrical stimulation (TENS) or relaxation techniques, can also be useful.

It's important to note that these three types of pain - inflammatory, mechanical and neuropathic - can coexist in the same patient, creating a complex clinical picture to manage. For example, a patient suffering from advanced osteoarthritis may also develop an inflammatory component if fragments of cartilage irritate the joint, or neuropathic pain due to nerve compression caused by joint deformity. Managing these types of pain therefore requires detailed assessment, so that treatment can be adapted to each type of pain and multimodal management can be proposed.

- **Non-drug strategies for pain relief**

Massage, thermotherapy, gentle mobilization, relaxation.

Massage, **thermotherapy**, **gentle mobilization** and **relaxation** are essential complementary approaches in the management of patients suffering from chronic pain and functional limitations, particularly in rheumatology. Each of these techniques contributes to relieving symptoms, improving mobility and offering an overall sense of well-being, while integrating harmoniously with medical or rehabilitative treatments.

Massage is a form of manual therapy that plays a key role in the management of muscle and joint pain. It relaxes contracted muscles, often associated with chronic pain, and improves local blood circulation, promoting tissue oxygenation and helping to reduce mild inflammation. By applying gentle, targeted pressure, the masseur or caregiver can also reduce muscle tension caused by compensatory postures, common in patients with joint pain. For example, a patient with osteoarthritis of the knee may unconsciously overload other parts of the body, such as the lower back or hips, leading to secondary pain. Massage relieves these areas of tension, while providing a sense of relaxation and general comfort. Massage is particularly beneficial for patients suffering from mechanical pain, but can also be used to soothe muscles in patients with inflammatory pain, provided the technique is adapted so as not to exacerbate the inflammation.

Thermotherapy, on the other hand, uses heat or cold to relieve joint pain and stiffness. Heat treatment, often applied in the form of hot compresses, heating pads or hot baths, is particularly effective in relaxing muscles and improving blood circulation, helping to reduce stiffness and increase joint flexibility. Heat is often recommended for patients suffering from conditions such as osteoarthritis, where worn cartilage makes movement painful and stiff. By increasing blood flow to muscles and joints, thermotherapy promotes better tissue oxygenation and helps flush out toxins that can contribute to local inflammation. On the other hand, cold, applied in the form of ice packs or cold compresses, is particularly useful for reducing inflammation and swelling during inflammatory flare-ups, as in rheumatoid arthritis or gout. Cold causes vasoconstriction, which limits the influx of inflammatory fluid into the joint, relieving acute pain and swelling.

Gentle mobilization is a crucial technique in the rehabilitation of patients suffering from rheumatic diseases. It involves slow, controlled joint movements, either passively (where the caregiver helps the patient to move without effort) or actively (where the patient participates in the movement). Gentle mobilization helps to maintain or improve joint amplitude, prevent stiffness and strengthen the muscles that support the joints. In pathologies such as ankylosing spondylitis, where the spine tends to become progressively rigid, gentle mobilization helps to preserve flexibility as far as possible, and prevent joints from locking into disabling positions. Although gentle, this technique also helps prevent muscle atrophy in patients who are immobilized or not very mobile. It provides continuous stimulation of muscles and joints, without overtaxing them or aggravating existing pain. As a complement to physical care, gentle mobilization helps patients maintain a certain level of autonomy and comfort in their daily lives.

Finally, **relaxation** plays a central role in the management of chronic pain and emotional distress associated with rheumatic diseases. Relaxation enables patients to reduce their stress levels, which often aggravate pain perception. Techniques such as deep breathing, guided meditation and positive visualization help to calm the nervous system, reduce involuntary muscle tension and lower the pain threshold. In rheumatology, relaxation can be used alongside other techniques to help patients better manage moments of crisis, by offering them tools to relax mentally and physically. Progressive relaxation, for example, in which the patient sequentially contracts and then releases each muscle group, helps to make the body aware of tensions and to release them. This practice helps to reduce anxiety, improve sleep quality and promote a general state of well-being, which is essential for patients suffering from chronic pain.

- **Involvement of the caregiver in medication management of pain**

Treatment monitoring, compliance, potential side effects.
Treatment monitoring, compliance and the management of **potential side effects** are essential components of rheumatology patient management. They play a central role in treatment efficacy and patient quality of life, particularly in chronic diseases such as rheumatoid arthritis, systemic lupus erythematosus and severe osteoarthritis. Careful, rigorous treatment management not only optimizes clinical outcomes, but also helps avoid complications linked to adverse effects.

Treatment monitoring involves regular, careful monitoring of the patient's response to the therapies prescribed. In rheumatic diseases, treatments often include non-steroidal anti-inflammatory drugs (NSAIDs), corticosteroids, immunosuppressants or biotherapies. Each of these treatments, although designed to control inflammation, reduce pain or slow disease progression, requires ongoing evaluation of its efficacy and suitability for the patient's individual needs. For example, NSAIDs, used to reduce inflammation and pain, need to be closely monitored for potential risks to the digestive system, notably gastric ulcers. Similarly, biotherapies, which target specific components of the immune system, must be administered under strict supervision to ensure that they do not excessively weaken the patient's immune defenses, thereby increasing the risk of infections.

The role of the nursing team, and particularly that of the caregiver, is fundamental in this monitoring. The caregiver observes signs of improvement or deterioration, such as reduced joint pain or swelling, or, on the contrary, the appearance of new symptoms such as fever or unusual redness. Working with the medical team, he can report any changes in the patient's condition, enabling doses to be adjusted or treatments modified according to individual responses. Monitoring also includes regular analyses, such as blood tests to check for the absence of serious adverse effects, including liver or kidney damage, which are common with certain immunosuppressive or anti-inflammatory treatments.

Therapeutic **compliance**, i.e. the patient's ability to follow treatment recommendations correctly, is another major issue in successful rheumatology care. Patients with chronic diseases are often required to take several medications over long periods, sometimes for life, and this consistency can be difficult to maintain. Forgetfulness, discomfort or side-effects can affect compliance. What's more, some patients, faced with an immediate lack of visible results, may be tempted to modify their treatment themselves, which can have serious consequences for their state of health.

The caregiver plays a key role in encouraging patient compliance. He or she can, for example, ensure that the patient understands the importance of following prescribed doses at regular times, while informing him or her of the expected effects of treatment, both positive and potentially unpleasant. By clearly explaining the long-term benefits of adherence to treatment, he or she helps the patient realize that stabilizing the disease, or reducing inflammatory flare-ups, depends on rigorous regularity. He can also suggest practical solutions to improve compliance, such as the use of pillboxes, medication reminders via mobile applications, or encourage therapeutic education sessions.

Finally, the management of **potential side effects** is a major concern in rheumatology treatment monitoring. Every drug, especially when used long-term, carries the risk of side effects, and it is essential to anticipate them in order to minimize them. For example, corticosteroids, although effective in reducing inflammation and relieving pain, can have significant side effects when taken over a long period, such as osteoporosis, weight gain, skin brittleness and increased risk of infection. Biotherapies, on the other hand, can weaken the immune system and expose patients to serious infections. In this context, it is crucial to regularly monitor the patient's health parameters, notably through blood tests or other medical analyses.

The caregiver, being in daily contact with the patient, is often the first to spot signs of side effects. They may observe symptoms such as stomach upset, unusual bleeding, excessive fatigue or signs of infection. By promptly reporting these symptoms to the medical team, adjustments can be made to avoid serious complications. For example, in the case of gastrointestinal disorders on NSAIDs, a gastric protector can be added to the treatment, or a biotherapy can be adjusted in the event of a significant drop in white blood cells, which would signal a weakening of the immune system.

Patient education also plays an important role in managing side effects. It is essential that patients are informed of potential side effects before starting a new treatment, so that they can quickly recognize warning signs. This enables early intervention and limits the risk of complications. The caregiver can reassure the patient that most side effects are controllable and temporary, while providing practical advice on how to manage them, such as adapting diet or implementing infection control measures.

Chapter 6

Technical care in rheumatology

- **Administration of specific treatments**

Infusions, subcutaneous and intramuscular injections.

Infusions, **subcutaneous injections** and **intramuscular injections** are essential modes of administration in the management of rheumatic diseases, particularly when oral treatments are insufficient or unsuitable for the patient's specific needs. These techniques enable drugs to be delivered effectively, often over the long term, and are crucial for controlling inflammatory, autoimmune or degenerative diseases such as rheumatoid arthritis, ankylosing spondylitis or systemic lupus erythematosus.

Infusions involve the intravenous administration of drugs directly into the bloodstream, usually via a slow infusion over a set period of time. In rheumatology, infusions are commonly used to deliver biotherapies, immunosuppressants, or treatments based on monoclonal antibodies, which specifically target immune system molecules responsible for inflammation. These treatments are often prescribed when oral therapies fail to control inflammation, or when the patient has severe forms of inflammatory disease.

The advantage of infusion is that it enables rapid, controlled diffusion of the drug throughout the body, ensuring rapid, effective action. What's more, due to the prolonged nature of these treatments, infusions are often administered at regular intervals, ranging from a few weeks to several months, helping to maintain a stable concentration of the drug in the blood. Infusions require careful monitoring during administration, due to the risk of allergic reactions or immediate side effects. The caregiver plays a key role in this monitoring, observing for signs of discomfort, redness or other abnormal symptoms in the patient, while ensuring that the infusion takes place under optimal conditions.

Subcutaneous injections, meanwhile, are another method commonly used in rheumatology to administer drugs, particularly biotherapies or certain immunosuppressive drugs. These injections involve introducing the drug into the fatty layer beneath the skin, where it is slowly absorbed into the bloodstream. They are frequently used in chronic diseases, as they enable regular, controlled administration of small quantities of medication over a prolonged period. For example, patients with rheumatoid arthritis may receive subcutaneous injections of biotherapies every week or two.

One of the advantages of subcutaneous injection is that it can often be carried out at home by the patient himself, after appropriate training. This allows greater autonomy and reduces the need to visit the hospital for each administration. Here, the caregiver has an essential role to play in the patient's therapeutic education, teaching good practices for self-administration of injections, ensuring that hygiene and preparation techniques are followed, and monitoring for any local reactions, such as redness, swelling or pain at the injection site. The caregiver can also provide psychological support, reassuring the patient about his or her ability to carry out these injections independently and manage any discomfort.

Finally, **intramuscular injections** are another widely-used route of administration, especially when the drug needs to be absorbed quickly or is irritating to subcutaneous tissue. This type of injection involves introducing the drug directly into a muscle, where it is rapidly absorbed by the blood vessels that irrigate the muscles. Intramuscular injections are often used to administer corticosteroids in the treatment of acute inflammatory flare-ups, as in rheumatoid arthritis or ankylosing spondylitis. These injections can offer rapid symptomatic relief, particularly in severe attacks where joint inflammation is intense and pain needs to be brought under control quickly.

Intramuscular administration is generally performed in large muscles, such as the deltoid (shoulder), vastus lateralis (thigh) or gluteal muscles. It requires a certain technique to avoid complications such as nerve or vascular damage, and the caregiver must ensure that strict hygiene and anatomy protocols are followed to guarantee safe injection. After injection, it is also important to monitor the patient for potential side effects such as excessive pain, inflammation of the injection site, or signs of infection.

Monitoring for side effects is a common feature of all these forms of administration. Each **method** - whether infusion, subcutaneous or intramuscular injection - entails specific risks, whether immediate effects such as allergic reactions, or more delayed effects such as infections, redness or persistent pain at the injection site. The caregiver, often in direct contact with the patient, is a key player in the early detection of these complications. By carefully observing clinical signs and maintaining regular communication with the patient, they can quickly report any problems to the medical team, enabling treatment to be adapted if necessary.

- **Monitoring treatment with biotherapies and immunosuppressants**
  Roles and precautions for caregivers in the face of infection risks.

Caregivers play an essential role in preventing and managing the **risk of infection**, particularly in patients with rheumatic diseases, many of whom receive immunosuppressive or biotherapeutic treatments that make them more vulnerable to infection. These patients, with their weakened immune systems, are at increased risk of developing opportunistic infections, whether bacterial, viral or fungal in origin. Caregivers' vigilance and precautions are therefore crucial to avoid these complications, which can lead to a worsening of the disease and compromise the effectiveness of treatment.

One of the caregiver's primary roles is to ensure the strict application of hygiene measures, both for themselves and for the patient. Adherence to basic practices, such as regular hand-washing with soap and water or the use of hydro-alcoholic solutions, is fundamental to reducing the risk of germ transmission. The caregiver must also ensure that the patient complies with these hygiene measures, especially in high-risk situations such as before meals, after using the toilet, or when wound care or injections are required. Simply reminding the patient of the importance of these gestures, by explaining them in an educational way, can help limit the spread of infectious agents.

Caregivers must also pay particular attention to the patient's **environment**. Regular disinfection of surfaces and medical equipment is essential to reduce the risk of infection. This includes frequently touched objects, such as door handles, telephones, or medical devices used by the patient. Care must also be taken to maintain strict cleanliness in areas **where** the patient is present, notably by ensuring that bed linen is changed regularly and that medical equipment is sterilized after each use.

Because of their treatment, immunosuppressed patients are more susceptible to respiratory infections, urinary tract infections and skin infections. It is therefore essential for **the** caregiver to **observe** the patient carefully for early signs of infection. These may include the onset of fever, chills, pain or redness in a wound, a persistent cough, sore throat or signs of unusual fatigue. For example, a mild fever that would go unnoticed in an immunocompetent patient may be the first sign of a serious infection in a patient on biotherapy or immunosuppressants. By spotting these signs early, the caregiver can alert the medical team and enable early management, which is essential to avoid a deterioration in the patient's condition.

Care administration, whether it involves infusions, subcutaneous injections or wound care, also demands heightened vigilance on **the** part of the caregiver. Technical gestures require rigorous asepsis to avoid contamination. Before each treatment, the patient's skin must be disinfected with a suitable antiseptic, and sterile equipment must be used. In the case of infusions or injections, it is important to monitor the injection **sites** for any signs of local infection, such as redness, swelling or abnormal pain. If any abnormalities are noted, the caregiver must immediately inform the medical team to prevent a more serious infection, such as septicemia.

Another important aspect of the caregiver's role is **patient education**. Immunosuppressed patients need to be informed of the precautions they need to take to protect themselves against infection. The caregiver can, for example, explain the importance of avoiding contact with sick people, especially in times of flu or viral epidemics. It's also important to make them aware of the risks of food-borne infections, by giving them advice on proper food storage and hygiene, as well as the importance of cooking meats properly and washing fruit and vegetables thoroughly. While these tips may seem obvious, they are essential for patients with weakened immune systems.

Finally, the caregiver must be **vigilant** about the patient's vaccinations, as some may be necessary to prevent serious infections, but others may be contraindicated due to the immunosuppressive treatment. For example, live attenuated vaccines such as chickenpox or yellow fever are generally not recommended for these patients. On the other hand, vaccination against influenza or pneumococcus is often recommended to protect against potentially serious infections. The nursing auxiliary, in collaboration with the medical team, must ensure that patients are properly informed and that they follow the vaccination recommendations appropriate to their state of health.

- **Preparation for specific diagnostic examinations**
  X-rays, ultrasounds, scans, MRIs and post-examination monitoring.

Medical imaging examinations, such as **X-rays**, **ultrasounds**, **scans** and **MRIs**, play an essential role in the diagnosis, monitoring and management of rheumatic diseases. These tools enable detailed visualization of bone, joint and muscle structures, and the detection of abnormalities that would not be visible on clinical examination alone. Each of these examinations has specific indications, and their combined use enables doctors to better understand the evolution of the disease and adapt treatments accordingly. The role of the caregiver is important on several levels: in preparation for the examination, in accompanying the patient and in **post-examination monitoring**, especially when more invasive procedures are involved.

rays are-X one of the most common imaging examinations used in rheumatology. They enable us to visualize bone structures and detect signs of joint deformation, fractures, osteoporosis or degeneration, as in osteoarthritis. X-rays are often used to assess the evolution of diseases such as rheumatoid arthritis, where the aim is to detect bone erosions or reduction of joint space. The caregiver plays a key role in preparing the patient, ensuring that he or she removes any metal objects that might interfere with the imaging, such as jewelry or watches, and reassuring him or her that the examination is painless and quick.

Ultrasound is used in rheumatology to visualize soft tissues such as tendons, muscles and ligaments, as well as the synovial membranes around joints. It is particularly useful for detecting inflammation, joint effusions or tendon lesions, especially in diseases such as ankylosing spondylitis or gout. Ultrasound is non-invasive and involves no risk of radiation exposure, making it the technique of choice for regular monitoring. The caregiver assists the patient during the examination, positioning him/her correctly on the table and ensuring that the area to be examined is clear. He or she also reassures the patient if he or she expresses any concerns about the examination, explaining that ultrasound is quick and safe.

Scintigraphy is a more specific examination, often used to detect diffuse bone anomalies or hidden inflammation that other techniques fail to identify. It is based on the injection of a radioactive product into the body, which binds to areas of high bone activity, such as sites of inflammation or bone repair.

Scintigraphy is particularly useful for diagnosing systemic inflammatory diseases, such as lupus or rheumatoid arthritis, by revealing areas of active inflammation throughout the skeleton. The caregiver plays a crucial role in preparing the patient before the radiopharmaceutical injection, ensuring that the patient is informed of the procedure and the precautions to be taken after the injection. After the scan, the patient may need to drink plenty of water to help eliminate the radioactive product, and the caregiver may be present to remind him or her of these instructions and monitor his or her general condition.

MRI (Magnetic Resonance Imaging) is a state-of-the-art imaging technique that allows detailed visualization of soft tissue, bone and joint structures without the use of X-rays. It is particularly valuable for detecting subtle lesions in cartilage, tendons, muscles or intervertebral discs. In rheumatology, MRI is often used to evaluate complex pathologies, such as ankylosing spondylitis or joint lesions in rheumatoid arthritis, when a more precise assessment of tissues is required. However, the examination can be a source of anxiety for some patients, due to the noise produced by the machine and the feeling of confinement in the MRI tunnel. The caregiver plays a vital role in reassuring the patient, explaining the steps of the examination, and ensuring that he or she is comfortable before the procedure begins. He or she may also be present after the examination to check that the patient is feeling well, as a slight feeling of fatigue or discomfort may be felt after spending a prolonged time in the machine.

Once imaging examinations have been carried out, **post-examination monitoring** becomes an essential step, especially after procedures involving the injection of contrast media, as in the case of scintigraphy or certain MRIs. The caregiver must ensure that the patient has no allergic reactions or undesirable side effects following the administration of these substances. This includes monitoring for signs of malaise, skin rash, shortness of breath or nausea. If a reaction is suspected, the caregiver immediately alerts the medical team for rapid management. It may also be necessary to remind the patient to drink plenty of fluids after certain examinations, to help eliminate contrast media or injected substances.

At the same time, the caregiver ensures that the patient is well informed about the next steps. This may include specific instructions based on the expected results of the examination, or advice on short-term medical follow-up. For example, if imaging reveals active inflammation or significant lesions, the patient may need to modify his or her treatment or undergo further tests.

Chapter 7

Functional Rehabilitation Assistance

- **Collaboration with physiotherapists and occupational therapists**
  Encouragement of mobility, use of rehabilitation equipment.

Encouraging mobility and **using rehabilitation equipment** are two fundamental elements in the management of patients with rheumatic diseases, as they help to preserve or restore joint and muscle function. Rheumatic diseases such as rheumatoid arthritis, osteoarthritis and ankylosing spondylitis often lead to a loss of mobility due to pain, inflammation or joint deformity. If left unchecked, this immobility can lead to increasing stiffness, loss of muscle strength, and a progressive decline in the patient's autonomy. That's why encouraging mobility and using appropriate rehabilitation equipment are priorities for caregivers, who are keen to maintain patients' independence as far as possible.

Encouraging mobility begins by gradually guiding patients through movements adapted to their abilities and state of health. Pain and chronic fatigue can discourage patients from moving around, but it's essential to explain that even moderate, regular activity can improve blood circulation, reduce joint stiffness and strengthen muscles. The caregiver plays a key role in this process, proposing simple exercises and reassuring the patient about the benefits of these movements. For example, he or she can encourage activities such as getting up regularly from a chair, walking a few steps with technical aids if necessary, or performing gentle stretches that respect the patient's joint limits. These gestures may seem minimal, but in the long term, they help maintain joint flexibility and prevent stiffening.

The caregiver's role is not limited to verbal encouragement; it also involves **active participation** to help the patient perform movements correctly, while taking care not to aggravate pain. This may include physical assistance when moving from sitting to standing, adjusting the patient's posture while walking or stretching, and using safe lifting or transfer techniques for patients with significant loss of mobility. The caregiver also observes the patient's reactions during these activities, adapting exercises according to pain tolerance and functional capabilities.

The use of **rehabilitation equipment** is another essential component in helping patients regain or maintain their mobility. This equipment is designed to support joints and muscles while facilitating movement, enabling the patient to rehabilitate without risking injury. Among the most common devices are walkers, canes, orthoses and wheelchairs, which help patients to move around independently while reducing the load on painful joints. The caregiver plays a crucial role in educating the patient in the correct use of this equipment. He or she must ensure that the devices are well adapted to the patient's morphology and needs, that they are adjusted to the right height, and that the patient feels comfortable using them in complete safety.

There is also **active rehabilitation equipment**, such as exercise bikes, treadmills or balance boards, which are used under the supervision of healthcare professionals to help strengthen muscles, improve balance and stimulate coordination. These devices enable patients to mobilize in a controlled manner, with personalized monitoring to avoid any risk of injury. The caregiver can be involved in this re-education by encouraging the patient to use the equipment regularly, in collaboration with the physiotherapists or occupational therapists who supervise the sessions. He or she can also help organize these sessions and motivate the patient to continue exercising consistently, highlighting the progress made and the long-term benefits.

In rehabilitation centers or even at home, the use of **suspension systems** and other equipment to relieve body weight during exercise is also commonplace. These devices enable even the most fragile patients to perform functional movements without bearing the full weight of their body, thus reducing pressure on joints and facilitating mobility. This enables progressive rehabilitation, while providing a safe environment in which to resume physical activity.

The importance of **consistency** in using this equipment and encouraging mobility cannot be underestimated. Regularity is the key to achieving tangible results in terms of flexibility, strength and autonomy. The caregiver's job is therefore to maintain the patient's motivation, supporting him or her in moments of discouragement, and adjusting exercises or the use of equipment as the patient's condition evolves. This may involve celebrating small victories, such as a smoother walk, a reduction in morning stiffness, or even a reduction in pain after a period of activity.

Early mobilization is also crucial. The earlier a patient is encouraged to mobilize as part of their illness or following surgery, the less likely they are to develop complications associated with immobility, such as pressure sores, muscle loss or joint ankylosis. The caregiver ensures that every opportunity for mobilization is exploited, working in collaboration with the rest of the care team to establish an individualized rehabilitation plan that takes into account the patient's abilities and goals.

- **Passive and active mobilization techniques**
    Practical approaches to aid functional recovery.

Practical approaches to aiding functional recovery are essential in the management of patients with rheumatic diseases or who have undergone surgery, as they aim to restore patients' mobility, strength and autonomy as effectively as possible. Functional recovery is based on a combination of adapted exercises, mobilization techniques and progressive re-education, taking into account the patient's overall state of health and the specifics of his or her pathology.

The first step in **functional recovery** is a precise assessment of the patient's residual abilities. This enables a personalized rehabilitation plan to be drawn up, setting both realistic and ambitious objectives, taking into account current functional limitations while aiming for gradual improvement. The caregiver, in liaison with the medical team and physiotherapists, plays a key role in observing the patient's daily movements, reactions to pain and effort tolerance. This observation enables us to constantly readjust rehabilitation approaches according to the progress made or obstacles encountered.

One of the most commonly used **practical approaches** is **passive mobilization**. In this technique, the patient's joints and muscles are mobilized without effort. It is particularly useful for patients suffering from joint stiffness, severe pain or prolonged immobility. Passive mobilization, performed by the caregiver or physiotherapist, helps to prevent muscle contractures, maintain a certain range of motion in the joints and stimulate blood circulation. For example, in the case of a patient with rheumatoid arthritis or osteoarthritis, knee or hip joints can be gently flexed and extended to prevent them locking into a fixed position. This technique, although passive, is crucial for maintaining joint flexibility and preparing the patient for more active mobilization as soon as possible.

Active mobilization, which often follows a phase of passive mobilization, is a decisive stage in functional recovery. Here, patients actively participate in their own movements, performing exercises under supervision. These movements are often simple at first, such as lifting a leg, bending an arm or turning the head. Gradually, as the patient gains strength and confidence, the exercises are intensified. The caregiver encourages and supports the patient during these exercises, ensuring that movements are carried out correctly to avoid any aggravation of pain or injury. Active mobilization is essential to strengthen muscles weakened by immobility, and to restore the muscular endurance needed for everyday movements.

Balance and coordination exercises are also crucial to functional recovery, especially in patients who have suffered chronic pain affecting their posture and stability. Simple exercises, such as standing on one leg, walking on a line or using a balance board, help to strengthen stabilizing muscles and retrain the nervous system to maintain correct posture. For patients with balance disorders, such as those suffering from ankylosing spondylitis or certain forms of osteoarthritis, these exercises are essential to prevent falls and promote a safer gait. The caregiver can be present during these sessions to ensure the patient's safety, providing physical support if necessary, and to encourage them to overcome their fears of falling.

The **use of technical aids**, such as walkers, canes or orthoses, is also a practical approach to supporting functional recovery. These devices enable patients to regain their mobility while reducing the load on damaged joints. The caregiver must ensure that these devices are correctly adjusted to the patient's morphology and level of mobility. In addition, he or she must ensure that the patient knows how to use these technical aids independently and safely, while monitoring progress over time. For example, a patient who starts out with a walker may gradually switch to a cane, indicating improved stability and muscle strength.

Muscle strengthening techniques are another fundamental aspect of functional recovery. After a period of immobility, muscles weaken and can even atrophy. It is therefore crucial to strengthen them progressively to enable the patient to regain his or her autonomy. This is achieved through targeted exercises, aimed at stimulating specific muscle groups while avoiding overloading the affected joints. For example, elastic bands or small weights can be used to gently strengthen arm or leg muscles. The caregiver can accompany the patient in these exercises, encouraging him or her to maintain correct posture and perform movements fluidly, without straining.

Finally, **respiratory and cardiovascular rehabilitation** is sometimes necessary for patients whose mobility has been limited for a long time. Light exercise, such as walking at a gradual pace or using an exercise bike, can help improve cardiovascular endurance and restore optimal lung capacity. The caregiver monitors exercise tolerance, ensuring that the patient shows no signs of exhaustion or respiratory distress, and encourages slow but steady progression to more sustained physical activity.

- **Adapting the environment to promote patient autonomy**
  Fitting out rooms, advising families on home care.

Room design and **home advice for families** are essential aspects in the management of patients with chronic illnesses or functional limitations. A well-adapted environment can greatly enhance a patient's safety, comfort and autonomy, while facilitating the work of the caregivers and relatives who assist them. Whether in hospital or at home, it is crucial to create a living environment that minimizes the risk of falls, facilitates mobility and encourages independence.

In a hospital environment, the **layout of the room** must be designed to facilitate movement and care. It's important that the space is clear enough to allow the use of mobility aids, such as a wheelchair, walker or cane. The layout of furniture, such as the healthcare bed, bedside table and chairs, must be optimized so that the patient can access them easily without having to move too far or get up too often. Height-adjustable and reclining healthcare beds play a key role in facilitating care and enhancing patient comfort. These beds make it easy to change position, relieve pressure points and prevent the formation of bedsores, while helping caregivers to avoid excessive physical handling.

In addition to the bed, the accessibility of equipment and personal items must be a priority. We recommend placing the items most frequently used by the patient within easy reach, such as the remote control, telephone, water, medication and emergency call devices. Grab bars fixed to the wall or sides of the bed can also help the patient to get up more easily and safely. These simple features reduce dependency and enable patients to retain a degree of autonomy.

For patients who spend a large part of their day in bed, it is essential to provide **technical aids**, such as ergonomic cushions, foot supports or anti-bedsore cushions, to prevent immobility-related pain and maintain good posture. Caregivers, in collaboration with physiotherapists, ensure that these devices are regularly adjusted according to the patient's needs.

When the patient returns home, it is just as important to **prepare the living environment** in such a way as to make daily life as smooth and safe as possible. Families need to be well informed of the adjustments that need to be made to ensure a safe and functional environment. The first aspect to consider is safety in the home, notably by **preventing falls**, which represent one of the main risks for people with reduced mobility. This means eliminating obstacles on the floor, such as slippery carpets, misplaced electrical cables or poorly positioned furniture. It's also a good idea to leave enough space for the patient to move around freely with a mobility aid, such as a cane or walker.

Grab bars installed in strategic places, such as in the bathroom, near the toilet, or along corridors, are also recommended for safe movement. In bathrooms, the installation of shower seats or stools can help patients wash safely, without the risk of slipping. Non-slip mats are essential, especially in wet areas. For patients who find it difficult to get in and out of the bathtub, it may be necessary to consider more extensive arrangements, such as the installation of walk-in showers or walk-in tubs.

The **patient's room** at home should be designed with the same care as in a hospital environment. If possible, it should be located on the first floor to avoid stairs, which can be a major obstacle to mobility. A medical bed at home can also be considered to facilitate care and offer greater comfort to the patient. In addition, the use of **emergency call systems**, such as connected bracelets or pendants, is highly recommended to enable the patient to quickly contact a relative or an emergency service in case of need.

It is also important to provide families with **advice on the day-to-day management of** home care. Relatives caring for the patient need to be informed about good practice in assisting with transfers, such as moving from sitting to standing or getting out of bed, without risking injury to themselves or the patient. Training courses or practical demonstrations can be organized by healthcare professionals to show safe lifting or transfer techniques.

As well as providing care, the caregiver also plays a key role in **educating families**. They guide them on the importance of daily physical activity to prevent joint stiffness and muscle deconditioning. Simple exercises adapted to the patient's condition, such as gentle stretching or short, regular walks around the house, are recommended. The caregiver can also advise on the correct use of technical aids, such as walkers or wheelchairs, so that the patient can continue to move around safely.

Finally, **the** patient's **psychological environment** must be taken into account. Returning home can be a source of stress or anxiety for the patient, due to the fear of falling or losing autonomy. Families need to be made aware of the importance of maintaining an encouraging and positive attitude, while respecting the patient's rhythm. A calm, reassuring and caring environment promotes not only physical recovery, but also the patient's mental well-being.

Chapter 8

Rheumatology emergencies

- **Frequent emergency situations in this department**
  Acute gout attacks, exacerbations of polyarthritis, severe infections.

Acute gout attacks, rheumatoid arthritis exacerbations and **severe infections** are frequent complications in the management of patients with rheumatic diseases. These episodes, often sudden and painful, require a rapid and appropriate response, as they can considerably affect patients' quality of life, worsen their general state of health and lead to long-term complications if adequate management is not put in place.

Acute gout attacks usually occur suddenly, causing intense pain, most often localized in the joints of the lower limbs, particularly the big toe. This pain is caused by the formation of uric acid crystals that accumulate in the joint, leading to severe inflammation. The joint rapidly becomes red, hot, swollen and extremely sensitive, to the point where even contact with a sheet can be unbearable for the patient. Gout attacks are often triggered by a diet rich in purines (red meats, seafood, alcohol), episodes of dehydration or certain medications.

The management of **acute gout attacks** relies primarily on the management of pain and inflammation. Non-steroidal anti-inflammatory drugs (NSAIDs) are often used first-line to relieve pain, sometimes accompanied by corticosteroids to reduce inflammation more rapidly. Patients should be encouraged to rest and immobilize the affected joint during the attack. Caregivers can play a vital role in ensuring that patients take their medication at regular intervals, and applying cold compresses to reduce inflammation. Outside of attacks, education on diet, hydration and weight management can prevent further attacks, helping to limit recurrences.

Exacerbations of rheumatoid arthritis represent another major challenge in the management of rheumatic patients. Rheumatoid arthritis is a chronic autoimmune inflammatory disease in which the immune system mistakenly attacks joint tissues, leading to persistent inflammation. During an exacerbation, joint pain intensifies, joints swell more, and the patient may experience prolonged stiffness, particularly in the morning. These flare-ups can be unpredictable and very disabling, making daily activities extremely difficult.

Management of **polyarthritis flare-ups** often requires adjustment of treatment regimens. Patients on disease-modifying therapies (immunosuppressants, biotherapies) may require a temporary increase in dose, or the addition of corticosteroids to control inflammation. In times of crisis, rest of the affected joints is important, but should not be prolonged at the risk of joint stiffness and muscle loss. Caregivers should encourage gentle mobilization as soon as possible, as well as the use of technical aids to avoid overloading affected joints. In addition, regular monitoring of inflammatory parameters and symptoms is essential to adjust treatments in a timely manner.

Emotional support during these exacerbations is also crucial. Patients may feel frustrated, even depressed, at the uncertainty of the disease and the sudden episodes of pain. The caregiver plays a key role in providing psychological support, explaining treatment options and emphasizing that, although these flare-ups are distressing, they can be controlled with appropriate management.

Severe infections are another major complication in rheumatic patients, especially those taking immunosuppressive drugs to control their disease. These treatments, while effective in reducing joint inflammation, also weaken the patient's immune defenses, making him or her more vulnerable to infection. These infections can take the form of pneumonia, urinary tract infections or skin infections, and can quickly become serious due to the weakened immune response.

When a **severe infection** occurs in an immunosuppressed patient, it must be managed immediately. Symptoms to watch out for include fever, chills, intense fatigue, persistent cough, or localized pain (as in the case of urinary tract infections). The caregiver, often at the forefront of detecting these signs, must react quickly by informing the medical team and ensuring that the patient receives appropriate care, including antibiotics or antivirals if necessary. Managing infections in these patients is complex, as it may be necessary to temporarily suspend immunosuppressive treatments to allow the immune system to fight the infection. However, this can also increase the risk of inflammatory flare-ups, requiring a delicate balance between treating the infection and controlling the underlying disease.

In addition to medical management, **infection prevention** in immunosuppressed patients is essential. This includes implementing strict hygiene measures, educating patients on the importance of vaccination (particularly against influenza and pneumococcus), and raising awareness of the need to avoid high-risk environments during viral epidemics.

- **What to do in a medical emergency**
Quick reactions, emergency calls, first aid.
The ability to **react quickly**, make the appropriate **emergency calls** and perform **first** aid is essential in dealing with critical situations in the care environment or at home. These skills enable them to act effectively in the event of a sudden deterioration in a patient's state of health, be it a medical complication, an accident or a life-threatening emergency. Often on the front line in such situations, the caregiver must be able to remain calm and reactive, while performing appropriate actions to stabilize the patient until help or a doctor arrives.

When an emergency occurs, the first step is to **react quickly** to assess the seriousness of the situation. This requires constant vigilance to detect early signs of deterioration, such as altered consciousness, breathing difficulties, chest pain, or signs of shock, such as extreme pallor, cold sweats, or a weak, rapid pulse. Careful observation of changes in the patient's condition, coupled with a knowledge of the patient's medical history, enables the caregiver to quickly identify when a situation is critical.

At such times, **panic management** is crucial. The caregiver must remain calm, so as to be able to make the right decisions quickly. Once the emergency has been recognized, the first action is often to alert the medical team or contact the emergency services. This **emergency call** must be made as soon as possible, as every minute counts in situations such as cardiac arrest, respiratory distress or haemorrhage. The caregiver must provide precise and concise information when making this call, indicating the patient's identity, the nature of the emergency, the symptoms observed, and the time of onset of the signs. These details will enable the emergency services to prepare an appropriate and rapid response.

While waiting for the emergency services to arrive, **first** aid is crucial to stabilizing the patient and, in some cases, saving lives. One of the most critical situations is **cardiorespiratory arrest**, where rapid reaction is essential. If the patient loses consciousness and is no longer breathing, the caregiver must immediately start cardiopulmonary resuscitation (CPR). This includes regular deep chest compressions to maintain minimal blood flow to vital organs. If an automated external defibrillator (AED) is available, it should be used as soon as possible to try to restore a normal heart rhythm.

In other cases, such as **respiratory distress** where the patient is struggling to breathe or is showing signs of asphyxia, the first action is to check the airway. If airway obstruction is suspected (e.g. in the case of choking), the caregiver may need to perform Heimlich maneuvers to clear the obstruction. If the patient's respiratory condition nevertheless deteriorates, it is important to place him/her in a sitting or semi-seated position to facilitate breathing, while monitoring his/her condition until help arrives.

In the case of severe **bleeding**, such as heavy bleeding after injury or surgery, the priority is to control the bleeding. The caregiver must apply direct pressure to the wound with a sterile dressing or clean cloth, maintaining this pressure until help arrives. If the bleeding is on a limb, raising it above heart level can also help reduce blood flow. These simple but immediate actions can mean the difference between life and death.

Another common emergency is **severe allergic reaction** or anaphylactic shock, which can occur following the administration of a drug, food or insect sting. Symptoms include swelling of the face or throat, difficulty breathing, skin rashes, and sometimes loss of consciousness. Faced with this type of reaction, the caregiver must act quickly by administering a dose of adrenaline with an auto-injector if the patient has one. It is then imperative to contact the emergency services immediately, as further medical monitoring and treatment will be required to stabilize the patient.

Finally, in less urgent but nonetheless critical cases, such as a **fall** resulting in a serious injury or fracture, the first course of action is to avoid moving the patient, so as not to aggravate the injury. It's important to secure the area and assess for pain and any signs of serious injury, such as limb deformity or inability to move. Calling for help is then essential to ensure specialized care.

In addition to performing first aid, the nursing auxiliary must also **reassure the patient** and his or her family, while maintaining a constant dialogue with the emergency services when they arrive on the scene. This ability to manage the emergency while remaining calm and providing clear information is essential to ensure smooth, efficient care.

- **Collaboration with other healthcare professionals in critical situations**
  Coordination with doctors, nurses and other specialized teams.

Coordination between doctors, nurses, care assistants and other specialized teams is essential to ensure comprehensive, efficient and high-quality care for patients, particularly in complex medical services such as rheumatology. Each healthcare professional brings specific skills to the table, and it is by working together, in a collaborative dynamic, that we can meet patients' overall needs while ensuring personalized follow-up tailored to their state of health.

The **nursing auxiliary** is often at the heart of this coordination, being in direct and constant contact with the patient. They act as a **link between the various teams**, and are a valuable source of information for doctors and nurses. Thanks to their close proximity to the patient, orderlies are able to observe important details that can sometimes be overlooked during medical consultations, such as subtle changes in the patient's general condition, the appearance of pain, fatigue or worrying symptoms. This observational role enables other members of the medical team to be alerted quickly, facilitating rapid and appropriate care.

Coordination with doctors is crucial to ensure proper management of treatments and therapeutic protocols. Doctors, who are responsible for diagnosing and prescribing treatments, often rely on the caregiver's observations and feedback to adjust care. For example, if a patient shows signs of reacting to a treatment (such as excessive fatigue or new symptoms), the caregiver can report these to the doctors, who will adjust the dose or modify the treatment accordingly. This fluid communication ensures that medical decisions are based on up-to-date, accurate information, and that the patient receives the treatment best suited to his or her situation.

Similarly, **collaboration with nurses** is essential, particularly in the day-to-day management of care. Nurses, in charge of technical care such as infusions, injections or wound care, work closely with orderlies to ensure that these interventions take place under the best possible conditions. The orderly may assist the nurse during certain procedures by preparing the patient, ensuring his or her comfort and monitoring his or her condition during and after operations. They are also responsible for reporting any patient reactions to care, such as pain, irritation or signs of infection, enabling the nurse to adapt care accordingly.

Coordination with specialized teams, such as physiotherapists, occupational therapists and dieticians, is also an important aspect of overall patient care. In rheumatology, for example, functional rehabilitation is a key aspect of treatment to preserve patient mobility and prevent joint deformity. The nursing auxiliary works alongside the physiotherapist, ensuring that patients are mobilized on a daily basis and that the recommended exercises are carried out regularly. This continuity of care between rehabilitation sessions maximizes the benefits of specialized interventions.

Similarly, **collaboration with occupational therapists** is essential to adapt the patient's environment to his or her functional limitations. Working closely with the occupational therapist, the caregiver ensures that the patient uses technical aids such as canes, walkers or orthoses correctly, and adjusts the layout of the room or home to promote greater autonomy. For example, he or she may be responsible for installing grab bars, placing essential items within easy reach or ensuring that safety devices are properly in place, thus contributing to the patient's safety and comfort.

Coordination with dieticians can also play a role in improving the patient's overall health, especially when the patient suffers from co-morbidities such as diabetes or obesity, which can aggravate rheumatic diseases. The caregiver can ensure that nutritional recommendations are adhered to, by monitoring the patient's diet and reporting any problems, such as loss of appetite, eating difficulties or unsuitable eating habits.

Finally, **communication between all teams** is essential to anticipate and prevent complications. Coordination meetings, written transmissions and regular exchanges enable each healthcare professional to have a clear vision of the patient's progress, and to adjust his or her interventions accordingly. For example, during transmissions between care teams, the caregiver shares his or her observations on the patient's state of health, highlighting elements that might require special attention, such as a change in behavior, uncontrolled pain or signs of deterioration.

This information is invaluable in ensuring ongoing care and avoiding disruptions.

Chapter 9

Therapeutic Education and Prevention in Rheumatology

- **The role of the caregiver in therapeutic education**
  How to explain treatments, exercises and care to patients
  to promote therapeutic adherence.

Explaining treatments, exercises and care to patients is a key step in promoting **adherence**. A good understanding of the objectives of care and the reasons behind treatments enables patients to become more involved in their own care, to follow medical recommendations more rigorously, and to feel greater confidence in the care team. The caregiver, as the person who works closely with the patient on a daily basis, plays a fundamental role in this communication, providing clear, appropriate and reassuring explanations.

When it comes to explaining a **treatment**, an empathetic and educational approach is essential. Many patients, especially those with chronic conditions such as rheumatoid arthritis or osteoarthritis, can feel overwhelmed by the complexity of their treatment, particularly when it involves several medications to be taken at different times. The caregiver should start by presenting the treatment in a simple, accessible way, explaining what each drug is used for. For example, saying that "this anti-inflammatory medication will help reduce inflammation in your joints and ease pain" is more understandable than launching into a technical explanation of biochemical mechanisms. It's also important to remind the patient why it's crucial to follow the treatment regularly, even if they don't feel an immediate improvement, explaining that some drugs take time to work or are preventive.

In addition to explaining the importance of treatment, it is also crucial to discuss **potential side effects**. Patients may sometimes stop taking their medication because of unanticipated or misunderstood side effects. The caregiver must therefore prevent these situations by calmly explaining that some side effects may occur, but that they are often temporary or manageable, and that treatment should not be stopped without consulting a doctor. Reassuring the patient that solutions exist to minimize these effects reduces the anxiety associated with taking medication and reinforces adherence.

Rehabilitation exercises also play a fundamental role in the management of chronic rheumatic diseases, and their importance must be clearly explained to motivate the patient to practice them regularly. For a patient suffering from joint pain, doing exercises may seem counter-intuitive. The caregiver must therefore explain in a simple but convincing way that these exercises are essential to maintain joint flexibility, prevent stiffness and strengthen the muscles that support the joints. For example, he might say: "These exercises will help keep your joints mobile and reduce long-term pain. The more you move, the less likely your joints are to stiffen." It's also important to show how exercises should be performed correctly to avoid injury, while emphasizing the idea that they must be done regularly to be effective.

Accompanying the patient on **exercises** is an excellent opportunity to encourage and build confidence. The caregiver can adapt the exercises to the patient's abilities and encourage him or her to progress at his or her own pace, while showing that every little effort counts. Patience and encouragement are key to ensuring that the patient feels able to take charge of his or her rehabilitation, even if it takes time.

As for **day-to-day care**, such as wound management, personal hygiene or the use of technical aids, it is essential to explain these in a clear and practical way. Patients need to understand why this care is important to their well-being, and how they can participate, wherever possible, to preserve their autonomy. For example, when applying wound care, the caregiver can explain in simple terms: "We clean the wound in this way to prevent infection and promote good healing." If the patient is capable of performing certain gestures himself, it's helpful to show him how to do it, supervise him, and encourage him to actively participate in his own care. This helps them to feel in control of their situation, which in turn encourages greater commitment.

Another crucial aspect in promoting therapeutic adherence is the **personalization of explanations**. Every patient is unique, with different levels of understanding and concern. Some patients may be very inquisitive and want detailed explanations of their illness and treatments, while others may be more reticent or anxious about knowing too much. The caregiver needs to adapt his or her speech to each patient, taking into account his or her level of understanding, emotional state, and communication preferences. Sometimes, using analogies or concrete examples can help make medical concepts more accessible.

Finally, to maintain long-term adherence, it's important to **involve the patient** in the decisions that concern him or her. The caregiver can encourage the patient to ask questions about his or her treatment and express concerns. This shows that the patient has an active role in his or her own care, and reinforces motivation to follow recommendations. The caregiver can also act as an intermediary between the patient and the medical team, relaying the patient's questions or concerns so that these can be taken into account when adjusting treatment.

- **Preventing joint deformities and complications associated with rheumatic diseases**
  Explain exercises for maintaining mobility and wearing orthoses.

Explaining mobility maintenance exercises and the use of **orthotics** to patients is essential to fostering their understanding and adherence to these practices, which are often indispensable in the management of rheumatic diseases and musculoskeletal disorders. Mobility maintenance exercises, like the wearing of orthoses, are designed to prevent joint stiffening, strengthen muscles, and maintain or improve the patient's autonomy. However, if the patient is to follow them assiduously, it is important to explain their usefulness, how they work, and their long-term impact on quality of life.

Mobility maintenance exercises are specific movements designed to keep joints supple, improve range of motion and prevent stiffness, which can quickly set in with prolonged immobility. These exercises are particularly important for patients suffering from chronic diseases such as osteoarthritis or rheumatoid arthritis, which lead to joint pain and reduced mobility. The caregiver should explain to the patient that these exercises are designed to be adapted to the patient's physical capabilities, and that although they may seem light or simple, they have a significant impact on the patient's ability to move on a daily basis.

It's worth explaining that these exercises help **lubricate joints** by promoting the production of synovial fluid, which reduces friction between joint surfaces. This reduces the pain associated with inflammation and prevents premature joint wear. For example, for patients with stiff knees, the caregiver can suggest simple movements such as extending and bending the legs in a seated position, explaining that these gestures help keep the knees supple. If the patient feels pain, it's important to explain that exercises should be performed at the patient's own pace, without forcing them, and that regularity is more important than intensity.

Another essential point to explain is that **gentle strength training** around the joints helps to stabilize and protect them. Even simple muscle-strengthening exercises help to support weakened joints and improve muscular endurance. For example, isometric exercises (where the muscle is contracted without movement of the joint) may be recommended for patients with intense joint pain. The caregiver can demonstrate these exercises and explain that by strengthening the muscles around the joints, the patient will be able to better protect them and better manage his or her pain.

To help the patient understand the importance of these exercises, the caregiver should **demonstrate** and practice them with the patient. He or she can show the patient how to perform the movements correctly and ensure that they are carried out without undue pain. Furthermore, by explaining that these exercises need to be integrated into the daily routine, the caregiver helps to create a habit, insisting that a few minutes of exercise every day can have a significant long-term impact on mobility and quality of life.

When it comes to **wearing orthoses**, it's important to emphasize that these devices are designed to **stabilize and protect** affected **joints**, while enabling a certain level of activity to be maintained. Orthoses, whether worn for the wrists, knees or ankles, help to relieve joint stress by better distributing mechanical constraints, and limiting movements that could aggravate pain or cause deformity.

The caregiver must explain to the patient that wearing an orthosis does not mean a loss of autonomy, but rather that it is a tool that allows continued movement while protecting the joint. For example, a wrist orthosis for a patient suffering from tendonitis or polyarthritis can reduce pain during repetitive movements, while allowing a certain degree of mobility. The orthosis acts as a support without completely immobilizing the joint, enabling the patient to maintain function while avoiding aggravating the condition.

It's also important to **demystify the wearing of orthoses** by explaining how they work and how they should be fitted. The caregiver can demonstrate how to put the orthosis on correctly, checking that it fits properly without being too tight, which could lead to circulation problems or excessive pressure. It is essential that the patient understands that an ill-fitting or badly worn orthosis can be counterproductive and cause additional pain.

The caregiver should also explain how **often** orthoses are to be worn. Some orthoses are intended to be worn only during physical activity to prevent excessive movement, while others can be worn all the time to stabilize the joint during the rest phase. Clarifying these aspects with the patient helps him or her to better understand when and why to use the orthosis, and thus maximize its effectiveness.

Finally, it's important to stress that wearing a brace is not a substitute for **rehabilitation exercises**. Orthoses provide temporary support, but mobility and strengthening exercises are essential for lasting improvement. The caregiver can encourage the patient to integrate both aspects into his or her daily routine, explaining that the combination of mechanical support (orthosis) and active strengthening (exercises) helps to better manage the disease and prevent joint degradation.

- **Raising awareness of daily gestures and adapting the home environment.**
  Advice on adapting daily life to physical limitations.

Adapting **daily life to physical limitations** is an essential process for preserving autonomy, improving quality of life and preventing complications associated with chronic diseases or functional disabilities. Whether due to joint pain, stiffness, muscle weakness or chronic fatigue, physical limitations can make certain daily activities more difficult, if not impossible, to perform without assistance. However, with the right adjustments and support, it is possible to make these tasks more accessible and maintain a degree of independence.

One of the first **pieces** of **advice** to be given is to **simplify everyday gestures**. By making the most common tasks easier, such as dressing, cooking or washing, patients can save energy and avoid exacerbating their pain. For example, when dressing, the use of easy-to-put-on garments, such as pants with elastic waistbands or shirts with zippers, can greatly simplify this task. Specific tools, such as long tongs for grasping objects or elongated shoehorns, can also limit painful movements. The caregiver can encourage the patient to organize his or her wardrobe so that the most frequently used garments are within easy reach, thus avoiding repetitive and tiring movements.

It is also important to **rethink** the **organization of the living space**. For people with reduced mobility, it is essential that their environment is adapted to reduce physical effort and minimize the risk of falling. This can include redesigning the kitchen so that common utensils and foods are within easy reach, or installing grab bars in areas where movement is difficult, such as the bathroom or toilet. A **shower chair** can make personal hygiene easier, while the addition of **non-slip mats** makes wet areas safer.

The layout of the home must also take into account the patient's specific **mobility limitations**. If possible, we recommend limiting the use of stairs by locating the most frequently used rooms, such as the bedroom, on the first floor. If this is not feasible, the installation of a stairlift or ramps can greatly facilitate movement. In all cases, it's a good idea to keep passageways clear of clutter and remove any obstacles that might impede circulation, such as carpets, cables or low furniture.

Managing fatigue is another essential aspect of adapting to daily life with physical limitations. Many chronic illnesses, such as rheumatoid arthritis or multiple sclerosis, lead to persistent fatigue, which further complicates the performance of daily tasks. The caregiver can encourage the patient to organize his or her day so as to alternate periods of activity with periods of rest, in order to avoid exhaustion. It's helpful to prioritize the most important tasks at the time of day when the patient feels most fit, while taking regular breaks to avoid putting too much strain on joints or muscles. For example, cooking a simple meal at a time of day when energy levels are higher can avoid the need to resort to less healthy ready-made meals, while maintaining a sense of autonomy.

The use of **technical aids** is also central to compensating for physical limitations and maintaining independence. Canes, walkers, wheelchairs and orthoses are invaluable tools for facilitating mobility and reducing joint pain when moving around. Caregivers must ensure that these aids are properly adapted to the patient's morphology and needs, and must encourage their use by explaining that these devices do not represent a loss of autonomy, but on the contrary, a means of preserving it in complete safety.

In certain situations, it may also be necessary to call on **home help services** for more complex or tiring tasks, such as housework, shopping or meal preparation. These services enable patients to concentrate their efforts on activities they can carry out themselves, while delegating more demanding tasks. This helps conserve energy for the activities that matter most to the patient, such as leisure activities or spending time with loved ones.

It is also essential to **maintain appropriate physical activity**, despite physical limitations. Movement is important to avoid muscle atrophy, improve blood circulation and prevent joint stiffness. The caregiver can encourage the patient to incorporate small physical activities into his or her daily routine, such as short walks with a mobility aid, gentle stretching or supervised muscle-strengthening exercises. These exercises should be adapted to the patient's abilities and performed on a regular basis to maintain mobility and strength. It's also important to stress that even moderate physical activity can improve psychological well-being by reducing stress and boosting self-esteem.

Psychological support is another aspect not to be overlooked. Physical limitations, whether temporary or permanent, can be a source of frustration, discouragement and sometimes depression. The caregiver must listen to the patient's emotions, encouraging them to talk about their difficulties and providing constant moral support. Validating feelings of frustration or sadness linked to loss of autonomy, while proposing practical solutions for living better with these limitations, helps reduce feelings of helplessness and gives the patient a more positive outlook on his or her ability to manage daily life.

Chapter 10

Caring for the elderly in rheumatology

- **Specific features of rheumatic diseases in the elderly**
Prevalence of co-morbidities, multi-medication management and frailty.

The **prevalence of co-morbidities**, the **management of poly-medications**, and the management of **frailty** are central issues in the care of patients with chronic diseases, particularly in rheumatology. In addition to their main disease, these patients often have other associated pathologies, such as cardiovascular disorders, diabetes, hypertension or respiratory problems. These co-morbidities increase the complexity of care, as they influence the evolution of the main disease and require fine-tuned treatment management. In addition, frailty, particularly in elderly patients, further complicates care by increasing the risk of falls, loss of autonomy and undernutrition.

The **prevalence of co-morbidities** is high in patients with chronic rheumatic diseases. For example, rheumatoid arthritis is often associated with cardiovascular disease, while osteoarthritis may coexist with diabetes or obesity. These co-morbidities can influence the way rheumatic disease is treated, as they increase the risks associated with treatment, modify drug tolerance and require constant adjustments to therapeutic protocols. For caregivers, it's essential to have an overall view of the patient's condition, so as to take into account all conditions simultaneously. This requires rigorous coordination between different specialists (rheumatologists, cardiologists, endocrinologists, etc.) to ensure optimal management of each pathology.

The **management of poly-medications** thus becomes a major challenge. Indeed, these patients often take several medications simultaneously to treat their various pathologies. These may include anti-inflammatories to control rheumatic disease, anticoagulants to prevent cardiovascular risk, anti-diabetic drugs, anti-hypertensives, and many others. This large number of drugs increases the risk of drug interactions, treatment confusion and serious side effects. For example, a patient taking anti-inflammatory drugs for polyarthritis may be at increased risk of gastrointestinal complications if he or she is also taking anticoagulants for another condition.

The caregiver, who often accompanies these patients on a daily basis, plays a key role in managing multiple medications. They must ensure that patients take their medication as prescribed, at specific times, and in the right doses. The use of pillboxes, reminders via mobile applications or tracking charts can be an effective way of structuring medication intake and limiting errors. It's also important for the caregiver to keep a close eye on the appearance of side effects, such as dizziness, nausea, bleeding or allergic reactions, which may be linked to a drug interaction. In case of doubt, he or she must quickly alert the medical team to adjust treatments.

In addition, it is essential to explain to the patient and his or her family why it is so important to follow prescriptions scrupulously, even if managing poly-medication may seem cumbersome or discouraging. Patients need to understand that each treatment has a specific role to play in the management of their disease and comorbidities, and that unsupervised adjustments can lead to serious complications.

Fragility is another fundamental aspect to be taken into account, particularly in elderly patients. It translates into increased vulnerability to physical or psychological stress, reduced recovery capacity and increased risk of complications, such as falls, loss of autonomy or undernutrition. Frail patients are often both physically weakened, with atrophied muscles and painful joints, and psychologically more vulnerable, further complicating their day-to-day management.

Caregivers must be particularly attentive to signs of frailty, such as muscular weakness, impaired balance, involuntary weight loss or difficulty in performing activities of daily living. It is vital to implement measures to reduce these risks and maintain the patient's autonomy as much as possible. This can include encouraging gentle physical activity, such as walking or adapted muscle-strengthening exercises, as well as the use of technical aids to prevent falls, such as walkers, canes or grab bars in high-risk areas (toilets, bathroom, etc.).

Preventing undernutrition is also essential in frail patients, as involuntary weight loss can lead to reduced muscle strength, increasing the risk of falls and worsening dependency. The caregiver must ensure that the patient adopts a balanced, protein-rich diet, with snacks between meals if necessary to compensate for any loss of appetite. If malnutrition has already set in, coordination with a dietician may be necessary to adapt the diet and incorporate nutritional supplements.

- **Care techniques adapted to the elderly**
  Gentle mobilization, fall prevention, special care for fragile skin.

Gentle mobilization, **fall prevention** and **special attention to fragile skin** are fundamental elements in the care of patients suffering from chronic illnesses, functional limitations or age-related frailty. These aspects aim to maintain mobility, prevent accidents in the home, and protect fragile skin tissue, thereby helping to improve patients' quality of life and prevent serious complications.

Gentle mobilization is an essential method for preserving joint mobility, preventing muscle stiffness and maintaining blood circulation, while respecting the patient's physical limitations. It consists of slow, controlled movements, often passive, performed with the help of the caregiver when the patient cannot move alone, or active when the patient participates in the movement. The main aim is to prevent contractures and muscle atrophy, while relieving tension without causing pain.

This mobilization is particularly indicated for patients who are bedridden, suffer from rheumatic diseases or have chronic pain that limits their movements. For example, simple movements such as bending and stretching the legs or arms can be performed daily to stimulate the joints and prevent stiffness. The caregiver's support ensures that movements are carried out safely and comfortably, adapting the rhythm and amplitude of movements to the patient's abilities. This reduces the risk of complications associated with immobility, such as thrombosis or loss of joint flexibility.

In addition to maintaining mobility, gentle mobilization also helps prevent **falls**, which are one of the main causes of serious injury among the frail and elderly. Falls can result in fractures, severe bruising or even permanent loss of autonomy. **Preventing falls** involves both a careful assessment of the risks in the patient's environment and specific measures to ensure safe movement.

One of the first aspects of falls prevention is to adapt the **patient's environment**. This means ensuring that living spaces are sufficiently clear to avoid obstacles, such as slippery carpets or poorly positioned furniture. Installing **grab bars** in critical areas, such as corridors, toilets or showers, makes moving around safer and reduces the risk of falling. **The** use of comfortable, non-slip **footwear** is another important factor in stabilizing walking and preventing slips.

Caregivers also play a crucial role in **educating patients** and their families about how to avoid falls. For example, they may recommend getting up slowly after prolonged sitting to avoid dizziness, or using a **walker** or **cane** to improve balance when moving around. Repetition of this advice, coupled with careful monitoring of changes in the patient's physical condition, can effectively prevent accidents in the home.

Fall prevention is not just about making the environment safer, but also about **strengthening muscles** and **re-educating balance**. Simple exercises, such as standing up and sitting down several times in a row, or walking in a straight line, can help strengthen stabilizing muscles and improve motor coordination. These exercises, often performed under supervision, are essential for patients with loss of muscle strength or postural instability, and can help limit the risk of falls in the long term.

Finally, **special attention to fragile skin** is crucial, especially in the case of elderly or bedridden patients. With aging or chronic illness, skin becomes thinner, more fragile and less elastic, making it more vulnerable to injury, irritation and infection. **Pressure sores**, for example, are a frequent complication in bedridden patients who are unable to move regularly. They form at pressure points where the skin is compressed against the bed or chair for long periods, cutting off blood circulation and causing skin lesions.

The caregiver must therefore regularly monitor the condition of the patient's skin, paying particular attention to high-risk areas such as the heels, elbows, sacrum and shoulder blades. To prevent pressure sores, it's essential to **regularly change the patient's position** by gently mobilizing him or her every two hours, and to use **ergonomic cushions** or **anti-sore mattresses** to reduce pressure on sensitive areas.

What's more, **proper hygiene** is essential to preserve the skin's integrity. The use of gentle, moisturizing, non-irritating toiletries helps protect fragile skin from irritation. After cleansing, we recommend applying moisturizing creams to keep the skin supple and hydrated, and carefully inspecting risk-at areas for any redness or irritation that could signal the onset of a pressure sore.

Regular hydration is also essential, as dehydration can aggravate skin fragility. A diet rich in proteins and nutrients, combined with good hydration, helps to maintain healthy skin and promote healing in the case of small wounds.

- **Supporting family carers in caring for their loved one at home**
  Collaboration with the family, explanation of care and advice to improve autonomy.

Working with the family, **explaining care**, and providing **advice to improve the** patient's **autonomy** are essential elements in the care of people with chronic illnesses or physical limitations. The family plays a crucial role in day-to-day support, and as a caregiver, it is essential to work in partnership with them to ensure continuity of care and enhance the patient's quality of life. This collaboration is based on clear communication, explanation of the care provided, and advice tailored to promote the patient's autonomy.

Collaboration with the family begins with regular, transparent communication. The caregiver must share observations about the patient's condition, the care provided, and the goals of the treatment plan, while listening to the concerns or observations of loved ones. The family is often the first to perceive subtle changes in a loved one's condition, such as signs of increased fatigue, loss of appetite, or difficulty performing certain daily tasks. By incorporating this information into the care process, the caregiver can fine-tune care to meet the patient's real needs.

It is also essential to recognize that the **family is an integral part of the care team**, especially when the patient is cared for at home. The caregiver must therefore take care to explain care in an accessible way, taking into account the level of understanding of relatives. For example, if basic care such as hygiene, dressing or feeding is involved, it is useful to demonstrate the techniques to be used in a way that is safe and comfortable for the patient. Showing how to mobilize a bed-ridden patient to prevent bedsores, or explaining the correct use of technical aids such as a walker, are concrete examples that help families feel more confident and competent in their support role.

Explaining care is vital to ensure that the family understands not only **what needs to be done**, but also **why** this care is essential. For example, in the context of pressure sore prevention, the caregiver can explain that regular repositioning of the patient helps to preserve skin integrity and avoid serious complications. By understanding the impact of this care on the patient's health, the family will be more inclined to follow the recommendations and integrate them into daily life. This explanation also answers some of the questions or fears that relatives may have about performing technical care, such as managing catheters or monitoring infusions.

The caregiver must also **reassure the family** in the event of complications or complex care, explaining in detail what is happening and what to do next. This may include monitoring for signs of infection, recognizing symptoms of deterioration, or explaining the side effects of treatment. For example, if the patient is on immunosuppressive drugs, the family needs to be informed of the precautions to be taken to avoid infection and the signs to watch out for, such as fever or unusual pain. The caregiver can provide explanatory cards or visual aids to make this information clearer and easier to remember.

In addition to explaining care, the caregiver plays an important role in **educating the family** about strategies for **improving the patient's autonomy**. Encouraging autonomy, even in simple tasks, enables the patient to maintain self-esteem and a degree of independence. The caregiver can advise the family on how to adapt the home environment to facilitate this autonomy. This may include installing grab bars in bathrooms, using shower chairs or toilet risers, or arranging spaces so that everyday objects are within easy reach. These adjustments enable the patient to continue performing certain tasks alone, without having to constantly seek help from loved ones, which is beneficial for his or her psychological well-being.

The caregiver must also teach simple **mobilization techniques** to help the patient move around safely, without the risk of falling. For example, he or she can show the family how to assist the patient from sitting to standing, or how to use a walker or cane correctly to support walking. Encouraging mobilization is crucial to prevent muscle atrophy and maintain joint flexibility. Relatives can then be trained to support the patient in these movements, while respecting his or her physical limits.

Another essential tip for promoting autonomy is to **encourage patients to take an active part in their daily lives**, even in symbolic ways. For example, when it comes to household chores, the patient can be encouraged to carry out simple activities, such as folding laundry, putting away light objects, or helping to prepare meals. These small actions help to maintain minimal physical activity and reinforce the feeling of contributing to daily life, which has a positive effect on the patient's morale.

It is also important to discuss **emotional support** for the patient with the family. Relatives play a key role in motivating patients to remain independent. By positively encouraging their efforts, however modest, and avoiding overprotection that could aggravate dependency, the family helps to reinforce the patient's confidence in his or her abilities. The caregiver's role here is to explain that patience and benevolence are essential if the patient is to feel able to face up to his or her limitations without becoming discouraged.

Chapter 11

The Use of New Technologies in Rheumatology

- **Innovative technologies for functional rehabilitation**
  Exoskeletons, virtual reality and other rehabilitation devices.

Exoskeletons, virtual reality and other **innovative rehabilitation devices** represent a major advance in the field of functional rehabilitation, particularly for patients suffering from rheumatic diseases, trauma or chronic physical limitations. These modern technologies offer tailored solutions for improving mobility, strengthening muscles, restoring autonomy and facilitating the patient's reintegration into his or her daily environment. Complementing more traditional rehabilitation methods, these devices stimulate patient motivation while making rehabilitation more interactive, effective and personalized.

Exoskeletons are external mechanical devices that assist the patient's movements, supporting or amplifying the motor capabilities of limbs affected by a loss of strength or mobility. These devices are particularly beneficial for people suffering from partial paralysis, severe muscle weakness or neurological impairment. As part of rehabilitation, the exoskeleton enables patients to perform movements they would otherwise be unable to perform on their own, such as walking, standing or climbing stairs. By reducing the effort required to perform these actions, the exoskeleton helps to progressively strengthen muscles, while improving coordination and proprioception.

One of the main advantages of exoskeletons is that they enable patients to **regain a certain degree of autonomy** and reclaim movements they thought they'd lost. This not only has a physical impact, by improving mobility and strength, but also a considerable psychological one. The ability to stand and walk, even with assistance, can restore a patient's confidence and motivate them to persevere with their rehabilitation. These devices are often used in specialized centers, but more and more portable models are being developed for use at home, making it easier to continue exercising outside the hospital setting.

Virtual reality (VR) is another emerging technology that is transforming rehabilitation. It uses immersive digital environments to stimulate the patient's motor and cognitive skills in an interactive and motivating setting. In a virtual reality rehabilitation program, the patient is immersed in an environment where he or she must perform specific tasks, such as grabbing objects, moving elements or moving around in a virtual space. These tasks, while playful, are actually designed to improve specific skills, such as balance, coordination, or upper and lower limb mobility.

One of the great advantages of virtual reality is that it enables **progressive, personalized rehabilitation**. Virtual environments can be adjusted according to each patient's needs and abilities, offering tailored, progressive stimulation. For example, in post-stroke rehabilitation, VR can help rework hand-eye coordination and fine motor skills by simulating activities of daily living, such as preparing a meal or writing. The immersive nature of virtual reality enables patients to become more involved in their exercises, making rehabilitation more engaging and less repetitive. This can increase session attendance and improve overall results.

What's more, virtual reality makes it possible to **precisely monitor and measure** patient **progress**, thanks to integrated sensors that record every movement. Caregivers can thus adjust exercises in real time according to the patient's performance, offering more precise and responsive rehabilitation.

In addition to exoskeletons and virtual reality, other **innovative rehabilitation devices** are increasingly being used to support patients in their rehabilitation. For example, **rehabilitation robots** assist patients in performing repetitive movements, essential for restoring limb mobility. These robots are particularly useful in the rehabilitation of arms and legs after a stroke or partial paralysis, where repetition of movements is crucial to recovery. The robots are able to adapt their assistance according to the effort made by the patient, enabling a gradual progression towards autonomous rehabilitation.

Functional Electrical Stimulation (FES) devices are also used to help strengthen weakened muscles. These devices send electrical impulses to the muscles, causing them to contract in a controlled manner. They are particularly beneficial for patients with neurological or muscular injuries, as they restore movements that the patient can no longer voluntarily control. For example, a patient who has suffered paralysis can use functional electrical stimulation to activate the muscles in his or her legs or arms, thereby improving blood circulation, reducing muscle atrophy and facilitating active rehabilitation.

Finally, **treadmills with body weight support** are another valuable tool for gait rehabilitation. These devices enable the patient to practice walking while partially supported by a harness, reducing the load on the joints and enabling safe balance training. They are often used by patients in the early stages of rehabilitation, after an accident or surgery, to relearn how to walk without the risk of falling.

- **Digital tools for patient follow-up**
  Electronic medical records, mobile applications for pain and mobility management.

Electronic medical records (EMRs) and **mobile applications** dedicated to pain and mobility management represent a veritable revolution in the monitoring and management of patients, particularly those with chronic illnesses or physical limitations. These digital tools enable more precise, continuous and personalized care management, while facilitating communication between patients and healthcare professionals. They help to improve the quality of care, optimize treatment and empower patients to manage their own health.

Electronic medical records are centralized platforms where all information relating to a patient's health is stored, accessible in real time and consultable by the various healthcare professionals. They bring together essential data such as medical history, diagnoses, test results, current and past treatments, and surgical interventions. This centralization of information gives doctors, nurses, physiotherapists and other caregivers an overview of the patient's state of health, facilitating care coordination.

One of the main advantages of **EMRs** is that they improve **continuity of care**. For example, if a patient suffering from rheumatoid arthritis consults several **specialists** - a rheumatologist, a cardiologist, an endocrinologist - each of them can consult the patient's complete medical history through the EMR. This enables co-morbidities to be managed more effectively, treatments to be adjusted according to other pathologies present, and potentially dangerous prescriptions to be avoided in the event of drug interactions. Caregivers, in particular orderlies, can also consult this information to adapt day-to-day care to the patient's specific needs. For example, if immunosuppressive treatment is prescribed, the caregiver will be able to reinforce infection prevention measures.

What's more, **EMRs** facilitate the **transmission of information** in real time. In the event of hospitalization or emergency consultation, caregivers can quickly access the patient's medical history without having to resort to paper files or fragmented information. This saves precious time and avoids errors due to miscommunication. EMRs also enable patient progress to be monitored more systematically, recording clinical evolutions and adjusting treatments where necessary.

Mobile applications for pain and mobility management are another digital tool increasingly used to improve patients' autonomy and quality of life. These applications enable patients to monitor their condition in real time, record their symptoms and receive personalized advice on how to manage their pain and maintain their mobility.

As part of **pain management**, these applications enable patients to record the intensity of their pain on a daily basis, the factors that aggravate or relieve it, and the effect of their medication. This data is then shared with healthcare professionals, who can adjust treatments according to the information provided. For example, a patient suffering from chronic pain associated with ankylosing spondylitis can record his or her pain levels after each dose of medication, enabling the doctor to know whether the treatment is effective or needs to be modified. In addition, these applications often offer relaxation or guided meditation programs, breathing exercises to relieve pain, or advice on positions to adopt to limit stress on the joints.

When it comes to **mobility**, mobile applications can offer personalized exercises, explanatory videos and reminders to encourage patients to carry out their rehabilitation exercises. They can also track progress in terms of range of motion, muscle strength and endurance. Caregivers can access the data collected by these applications to monitor the regularity and effectiveness of exercises, and adapt rehabilitation programs according to the patient's needs.

Some applications even integrate **motion sensors** or wearable devices, such as connected watches, to measure the patient's movements, analyze gait, and detect any imbalances or risks of falling. This data can be transmitted to caregivers or relatives in real time, enabling rapid intervention in the event of a problem.

These applications also have a positive impact on patient **autonomy**, giving them an active role in managing their disease. The patient is no longer simply a passive recipient of care, but becomes a key player in his or her own care. By recording their symptoms, following their exercises and complying with medical reminders, they are better able to understand their condition and make informed decisions with their healthcare team.

The caregiver can also encourage the use of these digital tools by **helping the patient** to get to grips with them, particularly for patients who are less comfortable with technology. He or she can demonstrate how to use the various functions, check that information is correctly recorded, and encourage the patient to be rigorous in using the applications to derive maximum benefit from these devices.

Finally, **EMRs** and **mobile applications** enable better management of **teleconsultations**. With medical records accessible online, doctors can consult essential information before a remote consultation, and adjust treatments according to data collected by the patient via the apps. This is particularly useful for patients living in rural areas or far from medical centers, who can benefit from regular medical follow-up without having to travel.

- **Ongoing training in the use of new technologies**
The need for regular training to use these tools effectively. The **need for regular training** in the use of digital tools, such as **electronic medical records (EMRs)**, **mobile apps** for health management, and other constantly evolving technological devices, has become inescapable in the healthcare field. These technologies have dramatically transformed the way care is delivered, and to take full advantage of them, it's essential that all those involved in care, including care assistants, nurses, doctors and other professionals, receive ongoing training. Regular training enables these tools to be used effectively, improving the quality of care and ensuring better coordination between care teams, while enhancing patient autonomy.

The **rapid evolution of** healthcare **technology** requires constant adaptation of skills. EMRs, for example, frequently evolve to integrate new functionalities, improve the user interface, and meet the need for coordination between different medical teams. Without regular training, healthcare professionals run the risk of not making full use of the capabilities of these tools, or of encountering technical difficulties that could slow down patient care. What's more, updates to these technologies may include important new features, such as new security protocols to protect sensitive patient data, making the need for training all the more crucial.

For **caregivers**, who are often in direct contact with patients and involved in the day-to-day management of their medical follow-up, it is imperative to understand how to **access EMRs, consult essential information**, and **pass on observations** to other members of the medical team. For example, a good command of EMRs enables caregivers to quickly report any worrying developments in the patient's condition, such as worsening pain or the appearance of new symptoms, enabling rapid intervention by doctors. In addition, training enables them to make better use of specific EMR functionalities, such as treatment tracking, appointment management, or direct communication with other healthcare professionals.

The use of **mobile applications** dedicated to managing pain, mobility and other aspects of medical monitoring also requires specific skills. Caregivers need to be able to understand the data collected by these apps, interpret it correctly, and use it to adjust care. For example, if an app indicates that a patient's pain has increased significantly at certain times of the day, the caregiver needs to know how to relay this information to doctors and adapt comfort care or physical exercise accordingly. Without proper training, this valuable data risks being under-used or misinterpreted, which could compromise the effectiveness of care.

In addition, **ongoing training** helps maintain a high level of **data security**, a crucial issue in the use of digital healthcare tools. Confidentiality of medical data is a priority, and every healthcare professional needs to be aware of best practices for protecting sensitive patient information. This includes using secure passwords, managing data access, and implementing recommended cybersecurity protocols. Regular training ensures that caregivers are up to date on these practices, which is essential to avoid data breaches and protect patients' rights.

What's more, proper training in digital tools enables caregivers to manage their daily tasks **more efficiently**. By mastering the functionalities of EMRs and mobile applications, they can reduce the time spent entering data, searching for information or organizing care. This frees up time to focus on direct patient care, improving the quality of care provided and strengthening the relationship between caregiver and patient. Automated management of alerts, medication reminders and notifications linked to changes in the patient's state of health becomes more fluid and less error-prone.

Continuing education is not limited to technical aspects. It also includes the **ethical and practical** aspects of using technology in healthcare. It is important for caregivers to understand the implications of these tools in their relationship with patients, and to know how to support them in the appropriation of these technologies. More and more patients, particularly the elderly or those suffering from chronic illnesses, are using mobile applications to monitor their state of health. Caregivers need not only to be comfortable with these tools, but also to be able to guide patients in their use, help them overcome their reluctance, and encourage them to take advantage of them to better manage their disease.

This also means that part of the training must be devoted to **providing educational support to patients**. For example, a caregiver needs to be able to explain to a patient how to use an app to monitor their pain, how to record the information correctly, and how to interpret the basic data to adjust their daily activity or treatment. Without a good understanding of these tools, patients risk becoming discouraged or misusing them, which could adversely affect their medical follow-up.

Finally, training also **strengthens collaboration between care teams**. By better understanding the tools used by different healthcare professionals, everyone can more easily coordinate their actions and ensure that important information is shared seamlessly. For example, data collected by a mobility monitoring application can be integrated into the electronic medical record and shared with physiotherapists, doctors and nurses, enabling more comprehensive and coherent care.

Conclusion:

The Future of Rheumatology and the Growing Role of the Nurses' Aide

- **New therapeutic approaches**
  Innovations in biotherapy, cell therapy and personalized medicine.

Innovations in biotherapies, **cell therapies** and **personalized medicine** are ushering in a new era in disease treatment, particularly for complex pathologies such as autoimmune diseases, cancers and genetic disorders. These revolutionary advances offer more targeted, more effective treatment options, better adapted to the specificities of each patient, based on an in-depth understanding of molecular biology, immunology and genetic technologies. They represent a major turning point in the way diseases are not only treated, but also prevented and managed.

Biotherapies, which include treatments derived from living organisms, such as monoclonal antibodies, cytokines or specific receptor inhibitors, have transformed the treatment of many diseases, notably autoimmune diseases such as rheumatoid arthritis, lupus and multiple sclerosis. Unlike conventional treatments, biotherapies act in a more targeted way, precisely modulating certain immune system functions, thereby reducing side effects and improving treatment efficacy. For example, monoclonal antibodies are designed to target specific molecules, such as TNF-alpha or interleukin-6, which are involved in the chronic inflammation observed in these diseases. By blocking these molecules, biotherapies can halt the inflammatory process at source, offering lasting relief from symptoms.

These biotherapies have also revolutionized cancer treatment, particularly with the advent of **immunotherapy**, which uses the patient's own immune system to recognize and destroy cancer cells. Checkpoint inhibitors, such as pembrolizumab or nivolumab, release the brakes on the immune system, enabling immune cells to attack tumors more effectively. These treatments, though complex, have shown promising results, with lasting remissions in some patients with previously difficult-to-treat cancers.

Cellular therapies represent another major advance in the field of medicine. These therapies involve using cells, often modified or grown in the laboratory, to treat or repair damaged tissue. One of the most emblematic examples is **CAR-T cell therapy**, used to treat certain types of blood cancer such as leukemia or lymphoma. In this approach, the patient's own T cells - immune system cells - are harvested, genetically modified to express a specific receptor (CAR, for Chimeric Antigen Receptor) capable of recognizing cancer cells, then reinjected into the body to destroy the tumor cells. This therapy, although complex and requiring customization for each patient, has shown spectacular results in cancers previously resistant to standard treatments.

Cell therapy is not limited to cancer. In degenerative diseases such as Parkinson's or multiple sclerosis, stem cell therapies offer interesting prospects for regenerating damaged tissue. Stem cells, which have the ability to differentiate into different cell types, are used to repair or replace diseased cells. For example, in Parkinson's disease research, stem cells are being experimented with to replace dopaminergic neurons destroyed by the disease, in order to restore patients' motor functions. Although these therapies are still in the experimental phase, they offer a glimmer of hope for patients suffering from hitherto incurable diseases.

These innovations are part of a broader approach to **personalized medicine**, which aims to tailor treatments to each patient's specific genetic, biological and environmental characteristics. Traditional medicine often adopts a "one size fits all" approach, with standardized treatments for groups of patients with the same symptoms. Personalized medicine, on the other hand, relies on a more detailed analysis of each patient's biological profile, enabling the most appropriate treatments to be chosen according to his or her unique characteristics.

One of the foundations of personalized medicine is **genomics**, i.e. the study of the patient's genome (set of genes). Thanks to genome sequencing, it is now possible to detect specific genetic mutations that predispose to certain diseases or influence response to treatment. For example, in the field of cancer, genetic analysis of tumors makes it possible to identify precise mutations that guide the choice of targeted therapies, such as tyrosine kinase inhibitors to treat cancers with EGFR mutations. This approach maximizes treatment efficacy while minimizing side effects, as drugs are chosen according to their ability to act on the specific mutation present in the patient.

Personalized medicine doesn't stop at genetics. It also takes into account other factors, such as the microbiome (all the micro-organisms living in the body), environmental exposure and lifestyle. This information is integrated to propose more global and individualized therapeutic strategies. For example, some patients may respond better to treatment by modifying their diet or physical activity to complement drug therapies, depending on the interactions between these factors and their biological profile.

Advances in **artificial intelligence (AI)** and **big data** are also playing a key role in the development of personalized medicine. By analyzing vast databases of patient data, AI can identify patterns and correlations that are not immediately apparent to doctors, enabling them to predict responses to treatment or anticipate the risk of complications. These tools make it possible to offer even more precise treatments, tailored to the particularities of each individual.

- **The changing role of the caregiver in rheumatology**
  More responsibility for patient management.
The evolution of care practices is increasingly moving towards an approach that gives **caregivers greater responsibility** for **patient management**, notably through more integrated, patient-centered models of care. Healthcare professionals, be they nurses, orderlies or other members of the care team, are called upon to play a greater role in coordinating care, monitoring patients and making day-to-day decisions. This trend is accompanied by a change in skills and a reorganization of practices, aimed at reinforcing

continuity of care and improving the overall efficiency of the healthcare system.

The **extension of caregivers' responsibilities** is largely based on the changing needs of patients, particularly those suffering from chronic illnesses or complex pathologies. These patients often require regular monitoring and ongoing management of their state of health, well beyond occasional medical consultations. By being in direct daily contact with patients, nursing assistants are on the front line in observing changes in their condition, identifying the first signs of complications, and proactively adjusting care. This proximity to patients gives caregivers a heightened responsibility to detect subtle changes that can have an impact on the patient's overall health.

One of the main responsibilities of caregivers is to provide **clinical monitoring** of patients. This monitoring is not limited to taking vital parameters such as blood pressure, temperature or pulse, but also includes observing symptoms, managing pain and detecting early signs of decompensation. For example, in the case of patients with chronic diseases such as rheumatoid arthritis, an attentive caregiver may notice a resurgence of joint pain or increased morning stiffness, signalling a flare-up of the disease. Thanks to this vigilance, the caregiver can intervene quickly by adjusting care or alerting the medical team, thus avoiding a worsening of the patient's condition.

This **increased responsibility** is also accompanied by more active participation in **treatment management**. Caregivers, particularly nurses and orderlies, are increasingly involved in medication management, both in the administration of treatment and in therapeutic patient education. They ensure that patients comply with their prescriptions, whether for taking medication, using medical devices or performing rehabilitation exercises. This involvement goes beyond the simple administration of treatments, as caregivers play a key role in monitoring **compliance** and evaluating the effectiveness of treatments. In the event of non-adherence to prescriptions, they are the first to identify obstacles and work with the patient to find solutions, whether this involves better organizing medication intake, explaining the benefits of treatment, or reporting undesirable side effects to doctors.

Therapeutic education is also a growing responsibility for caregivers. With the growing complexity of treatments and home care, caregivers are called upon to educate patients and their families on how best to manage their disease. This includes explanations on the use of medical devices (such as inhalers, insulin devices or orthoses), advice on lifestyle adjustments (diet, physical activity) and recommendations on day-to-day symptom management. By providing this information, caregivers enable patients to become more autonomous in managing their condition, while ensuring that care at home runs smoothly and safely.

Care coordination is another area where caregivers' responsibilities have expanded. In a context where patients are often followed by several specialists, be they doctors, physiotherapists, dieticians or occupational therapists, caregivers play a crucial role in linking the different teams. They ensure that each professional has the information they need to provide appropriate, coordinated care. For example, a care assistant may be in charge of transmitting information between the medical team and the physiotherapists, so as to adjust rehabilitation exercises in line with changes in the patient's pain or mobility. This coordination ensures that the interventions of the various healthcare professionals are harmonized, avoiding fragmented care or contradictory prescriptions.

Teleconsultation and digital tools, such as electronic medical records and monitoring applications, have also broadened the scope of caregivers' responsibilities. With these technologies, caregivers are able to continuously monitor patients, even from a distance. They can monitor health data in real time, such as blood glucose levels for diabetic patients or blood pressure fluctuations for those suffering from hypertension, and report any suspicious changes to doctors. This remote monitoring enables proactive management of chronic diseases and rapid intervention when needed.

Prevention also plays a central role in these new responsibilities. Caregivers no longer simply react to symptoms or complications, but actively participate in the prevention of health problems. This may involve promoting vaccination, raising awareness of the importance of regular physical activity, or detecting the first signs of undernutrition, dehydration or cognitive impairment in elderly patients. By adopting a more preventive approach, caregivers help reduce avoidable hospitalization, limit the progression of chronic diseases and improve patients' quality of life.

Against this backdrop of **increasing responsibilities**, it is vital that caregivers benefit from **ongoing training**. Rapidly evolving practices, medical technologies and therapeutic protocols require regular updating of skills to keep abreast of best practices and innovations in care. This ongoing training enables caregivers to better understand patients' specific needs, acquire advanced technical skills, and deepen their knowledge of how to manage complex treatments or emergency situations.

- **Conclusion: The vocation of the rheumatology orderly**
  A job for the heart, at the service of patients.

The nursing profession is above all a **profession of the heart**, deeply rooted in humanity, compassion and dedication. Being at the **service of patients** means much more than providing technical care or administering treatments; it means being present at every stage of their health journey, offering caring accompaniment, emotional support and ongoing attention to their physical and moral well-being. This role, often discreet but essential, is based on a relationship of trust, listening and empathy that is forged day after day with patients.

This profession demands a special kind of **human contact**. Caregivers are in direct contact with patients, often at times of great vulnerability: illness, pain, loss of autonomy, or isolation. At such times, the **human dimension** of the job becomes central. An attentive look, a reassuring gesture, or a soothing word can have a profound impact on a patient's morale, far beyond the scope of the medical care itself. It is this human contact, imbued with warmth and respect, that makes the nursing profession unique.

The **daily routine of a caregiver** is punctuated by gestures of attention and support, whether it's helping a patient to get up, feeding them, accompanying them in their rehabilitation exercises or ensuring their comfort. Every task, no matter how simple, is carried out with an eye to meeting the patient's individual needs, taking into account not only their physical limitations but also their emotional state. This work requires a great deal of **listening**, as each patient is unique in his or her expectations, fears and pain. You need to know how to adapt, find the right rhythm, and sometimes offer a listening ear to those who need to talk about their anxieties or loneliness.

In this sense, the caregiver embodies a permanent **psychological support**, capable of comforting and encouraging, especially when illness or dependence weighs heavily on the patient's morale. They are often the first to perceive signs of fatigue, discouragement or psychological suffering, and their role then goes beyond that of a simple carer to become that of a **companion**, ready to restore confidence and hope to those going through difficult times. Patients, faced with the fragility of their condition, find in the caregiver a reassuring presence, someone who is there, without judgment, to support them on their journey.

Being a caregiver also means **knowing how to adapt** to the challenges that each patient presents. Some patients face chronic pain, others a progressive loss of autonomy, while still others have to cope with disabilities that disrupt their daily lives. Caregivers must find the best solutions to improve their comfort and quality of life, working with medical teams to adjust care, using appropriate technical aids or encouraging simple gestures that enable patients to regain a measure of autonomy. This **ability to adapt** is essential in a profession where every day presents different challenges, and where each patient requires an individualized approach.

Being at the **service of patients** also means being present in moments of life often marked by **dignity** and **fragility**. Faced with illness or dependency, it is sometimes difficult for patients to accept help from others, especially when very personal tasks are involved. Caregivers must therefore show **respect**, **discretion** and **tact** to preserve the patient's dignity, reminding them that they are not defined by their illness or incapacity. This respect for the individual, his or her privacy, and autonomy, however limited, is at the heart of the caregiver's mission.

The caregiver is also a **valuable link** between patients and the rest of the healthcare team. They pass on crucial information on changes in patients' state of health, their needs, their pain or their difficulties, enabling treatments to be adjusted and overall care to be improved. This **coordination** between the various teams is essential to ensure that the care provided is tailored to the patient's needs and expectations. The caregiver thus becomes a key player in the continuity of care, acting both as a relay of information and a guarantor of patient well-being.

In this heartfelt profession, patient **recognition** is often a great source of motivation. Although sometimes silent or discreet, this recognition manifests itself in a smile, a thank-you, or simply in the fact that the patient feels safe and understood. For the caregiver, these small moments of gratitude reflect the importance of their role, a reminder that every gesture counts and that their work has a real impact on the lives of the people they care for.

In short, the nursing profession is a **profession of the heart**, where humanity, benevolence and compassion are at the heart of daily action. **Serving patients** means offering much more than technical care: it means being a constant support, a reassuring presence, and an attentive companion throughout the entire healthcare process. This demanding but deeply rewarding profession is based on listening, respect and dedication to improving the quality of life of those in vulnerable situations. It is this essential and irreplaceable human dimension that makes this profession so much more than just a job, but a true vocation.